Lower Limb Amputation

A Guide to Living a Quality Life

By

Adrian Cristian, M.D.

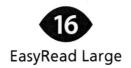

16

EasyRead Large

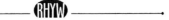

Copyright Page from the Original Book

Demos Medical Publishing, LLC, 386 Park Avenue South, New York, New York 10016. Visit our website at www.demosmedpub.com.

Library of Congress Cataloging-in-Publication Data

Cristian, Adrian, 1964-
  Lower limb amputation : a guide to living a quality life / Adrian Cristian. — 1st ed.
     p. cm.
  Includes bibliographical references.
  ISBN 1-932603-24-7
  1. Leg—Amputation—Popular works. I. Title.
  RD560.C75 2005
  617.5'8—dc22

                                                    2005008843

The purpose of this book is to provide information to readers so that they can make more informed decisions about their own healthcare. It should not be construed as medical advice and readers should always consult with their doctors.

COPYEDITOR: Jessica Bryan
PRODUCTION/TYPESETTER: Patricia Wallenburg, TypeWriting
PRINTER: Transcontinental
INDEXER: Joann Woy, Freelance Editorial Services
COVER DESIGNER: James Reyman, Reyman Studio

Made in Canada

ReadHowYouWant partners with publishers to provide books for ALL Kinds of Readers. For more information about Becoming A RHYW Registered Reader and to find more titles in your preferred format, visit:

www.readhowyouwant.com

TABLE OF CONTENTS

Adrian Cristian, M.D.
Assistant Professor, Rehabilitation Medicine
Mount Sinai School of Medicine
and
Chief, Physical Medicine and Rehabilitation
Bronx VA Medical Center
New York, New York

To Eliane, Alexander, and Chloe—the joys of my life.

Preface

Each year, several hundred thousand people in the United States undergo amputation surgery, most commonly as the result of diabetes or peripheral vascular disease.

This book deals with the many issues that amputees commonly face in the first year following their lower limb amputation, but also provides helpful advice for those who have had their amputation for a longer period of time, as well as for family members and friends.

The first six chapters deal with the causes of lower limb amputation, various types of amputation surgeries, and the postoperative/early rehabilitation phases of treatment. This is followed by a discussion of prosthetic components and the common problems faced in using a prosthesis; the special needs of children, older adults, and bilateral amputees; exercise and sports participation; and general coping skills.

Learning to live with a lower limb amputation is a great personal challenge. This book offers guidance, advice, and hope on how to live and thrive as an amputee.

Adrian Cristian, M.D.

ACKNOWLEDGMENTS

This book would not have been possible without the guidance, advice, and support of the following individuals: Eliane Cristian, M.A., Harriet Zuller, B.A., Richard Frieden, M.D., John W. Michael, M.Ed., C.P.O., James Klein, John Milani, C.P.O., and Diana M. Schneider, Ph.D.

CHAPTER 1

Introduction

If you are reading this book, you, a loved one, or a friend has probably had a lower limb amputation. You are not alone. Each year, several hundred thousand people in the United States undergo amputation surgery and must deal with the same issues.

This book is meant to be a comprehensive resource for both the new amputee as well as the individual who has lived with an amputation for several years. It is also meant to be used as a reference by family members who wish to learn more about caring for someone with an amputated lower limb.

The following overview discusses the key points in the book.

RISK FACTORS FOR AMPUTATION

The vast majority of lower limb amputations result from the complications of diabetes and/or peripheral vascular disease (PVD). PVD is the medical term for poor blood circulation in the arteries of the legs. Without adequate blood circulation, the tissues do not receive enough oxygen and nutrition to carry out their daily functions and are damaged as a result. Other risk factors associated with amputation include smoking, trauma resulting from accidents, and cancer.

LEVEL OF AMPUTATION AND POST-SURGICAL RECOVERY

There are several different levels at which the surgeon can amputate a limb. The most common are:

- Through the foot

- Ankle (Syme)

- Below the knee (transtibial)

- Through the knee (knee disarticulation)

- Above the knee (transfemoral)

The level of amputation depends on where there is the greatest blood flow and, therefore, the greatest possibility of healing. The surgeon often attempts to save the knee, because the energy cost of walking with an intact knee is much less than without it. The most common problems during the immediate post-surgery period are wound healing, infections, limited range of motion, swelling, and pain in the residual limb. The goals of this part of recovery are adequate healing of the residual limb, optimizing nutrition, minimizing pain and swelling, and slowly starting the rehabilitation process.

REHABILITATION

Given the complexity of care associated with the loss of a limb, you will probably spend time on a rehabilitation unit, where a team of health care professionals led by a physician will care for you. *Pre-prosthetic training* refers to the period of time between the surgery and when you receive a prosthesis. This training consists of exercises meant to improve your strength, stamina, and the flexibility of your body in anticipation of learning to use the prosthesis. Attempts will also be made to reduce the swelling of the residual limb using bandages and tight socks known as *shrinkers.*

THE PROSTHESIS

The minimum criteria needed to be fitted with a prosthesis include a healed residual limb, good balance, good strength, and the ability to hop with a walker for about 50 feet. A prosthesis is made up of several different components:

- Suspension system—needed to suspend the prosthesis from the body

- Socket—the shell that is in immediate contact with the residual limb

- Shank—the metal piece that connects the socket to the prosthetic knee or foot

- Knee component (for an above the knee prosthesis)

- Prosthetic foot

Initially, you will receive a temporary prosthesis, which will enable you to learn how to walk with an artificial limb. Approximately 6 to 12 months after receiving the temporary prosthesis, you will be ready for a permanent prosthesis that will last for several years. The decision as to which components are right for you depends on your medical condition, balance, and strength, and how you plan to use the prosthesis. Your physician, prosthetist, and physical therapist will help you in selecting the prosthesis that is right for you.

WALKING WITH A PROSTHESIS

Walking with a prosthesis can be very challenging. It requires a considerable amount of balance, stamina, and strength. A physical therapist will teach you how to walk with the prosthesis on different surfaces, utilizing a variety of assistive devices as needed.

COMMON PROBLEMS AFTER DISCHARGE FROM REHABILITATION

The most common problems experienced by lower limb amputees are those typically associated with an ill-fitting prosthesis, leading to skin irritation, superficial skin infections, and pain. Good hygiene is very important for lower limb amputees. The residual limb, socks, and gel liners should be cleaned every day. Pain is also very common in amputees. It could be in the residual limb itself or in other parts of the body, such as the lower back, knees, and hips. It is also common to have pain where the amputated leg used to be. This is known as *phantom pain.*

PREVENTING FALLS IN THE HOME

Living with a lower limb amputation places you at a greater risk of falling. In order to minimize your risk in the home, it is a good idea to remove loose rugs, clean up cluttered areas, and have adequate lighting in commonly traveled areas. Grab bars and a tub bench in your bathroom can help make this high-risk part of your home safer.

Minimizing the Risk for Additional Amputations

Having a lower limb amputation due to complication of peripheral vascular disease or diabetes can significantly increase your risk for future lower limb amputations, and it is important to protect your remaining foot. This can be accomplished by avoiding high-risk activities, such as walking barefoot. Also, investing in a good pair of walking shoes with a wide and high toebox can provide good protection for the fragile foot. It is also important to keep your foot dry and avoid using sharp objects on it. Have a foot specialist *(podiatrist)* evaluate the foot on a regular basis if you are a diabetic.

CHALLENGES FACED BY THE OLDER FRAIL AMPUTEE

Impaired balance, poor vision, multiple medical problems, and loss of strength and stamina all pose special challenges for older, frail persons living with a lower limb amputation. A slower-paced rehabilitation program with safety precautions, and prosthetic components that emphasize safety, stability, and ease of application, can be of great help.

THE CHALLENGE OF BILATERAL AMPUTATION

Living with two lower limb amputations requires a considerable amount of trunk control, stamina, and strength in the arms. It is more difficult to walk for long distances because of the high energy cost of walking with two prostheses. Some bilateral amputees opt for short, functional prostheses known as *stubbies.*

CHALLENGES FACED BY CHILDREN WITH LOWER LIMB AMPUTATION

The most common reasons for a lower limb amputation in children are birth defects, trauma, and cancer. Children are very quick learners and have lots of energy. They often adapt to prosthetic use faster than adults. Nevertheless, issues associated with acceptance by their families and peers can make prosthetic use more challenging.

SPORTS AND EXERCISE

People living with lower limb amputations are able to exercise and compete in sports because of advances in prosthetic design. Prosthetic components such as the knee and foot are usually lighter and have an array of different movement capabilities. Although there are certain inherent risks in exercising, these risks can be minimized with proper precautions.

COPING SKILLS FOR LIFE AFTER AMPUTATION

There is no "right way" to feel after the loss of a limb. Emotions are often tied to the cause of the amputation. Nevertheless, having a positive outlook, being pro-active about your care, and surrounding yourself with a good support system can be a big help.

People living with an amputation are not all the same. The reasons for amputation vary from individual to individual. Each amputee has different needs and a lifestyle that make his situation unique. The common denominator for all amputees, however, is the desire to function at the highest level possible. The goal of this book is to help people living with amputation to achieve their highest potential. Well-informed, knowledgeable individuals with amputations are able to take better care of themselves and are more effective self-advocates.

CHAPTER 2

The Causes of Lower Limb Amputation

Perhaps you are an older person who has had diabetes for many years, and you have been grappling with the problems associated with this illness, such as poor sensation and circulation in your feet. You may have already undergone a heart bypass surgery for clogged arteries.

One day you go to the beach and accidentally step on a sharp object, and then develop an infection in your foot. In spite of taking antibiotics at home, the infection gets worse, and your doctor admits you to the hospital for testing and antibiotic treatment. Eventually, a surgeon tells you that your leg must be amputated to save you from a life-threatening infection. Your immediate concern is to get through the operation, but you also wonder if you will be able to walk with an artificial limb. How will the loss of the limb impact your freedom, your ability to drive, and your ability to manage by yourself? You hope that you will not be a burden to your family or friends.

Perhaps you have been treated for poor circulation in your feet for several years. One day your foot becomes cold and blue, and you are rushed to the hospital for tests. A surgeon says that you will need surgery to bypass blocked arteries in your leg. After you undergo surgery, complications ensue and you need an additional surgery ... and then another ... until, finally, the surgeon tells you that he will have to amputate some of your toes ... and then a part of your foot; eventually he tells you he needs to perform an amputation above the knee. Meanwhile, months of being in and out of the hospital have left you feeling weak, and you have pain in the remaining part of your leg. You wonder how you will learn to use an artificial limb, and whether you will be able to return to your home, which has two flights of stairs. You wonder if you will ever be able to play golf again.

Maybe you are a young construction worker with a wife and two small children, and you sustain a severe injury on the job. You are brought to the local hospital where a surgeon tells you that you will lose your leg. At first, you may be in total disbelief because you have always enjoyed good health. Then you start to worry about how the amputation will affect your ability to support your family and play with your kids. You worry about whether your spouse will still find you attractive.

You may be a teenager who is diagnosed with bone cancer, and the doctor tells you that your leg must be amputated. You were doing well in school and had many friends, but suddenly your life has changed. Not only have you been told that you have cancer, but you are going to lose your leg as well. You wonder what your friends will think of you. You wonder if you will still be able to play sports.

The loss of a leg is a significant life-altering event. Although each of the above scenarios is different, they have in common the difficulties that are faced by anyone who loses a limb. These difficulties may include very practical concerns about managing everyday life, such as walking, shopping, driving, or going to school. They may also be more psychological in nature, in that amputation changes the way people see themselves, their relationships, and their future.

By far, the most common cause of amputation in the United States is from complications related to poor blood circulation and infection in the legs. People with diabetes are especially at risk for amputation. The sensation in the feet may be diminished, which may impair the ability to detect an injury when one occurs. Additionally, there may be fragile blood vessels that can be injured easily. The combination of poor sensation and poor circulation makes it more difficult to overcome an infection, and an infection in the leg may place your life in jeopardy.

Another cause of amputation is cancer of the bone. Typically, this occurs in children and adolescents. A child may have pain in the leg, usually around the knee, and an X-ray may show some abnormal bone formation. Amputation surgery is necessary to prevent the cancer from spreading to other parts of the body.

A child may also be born with one or more limbs that are small and deformed because of inadequate development prior to birth. The child may possess normal intelligence or have other developmental problems as well.

Another cause of amputation is trauma following an accident, or an injury sustained during military service in which the limb sustains multiple injuries to the bones, muscles, and blood vessels, making surgical repair impossible.

PERIPHERAL VASCULAR DISEASE

Peripheral vascular disease (PVD) can affect multiple blood vessels throughout the body. PVD is characterized by deposits of cholesterol and other substances in the walls of blood vessels, which affect the flow of blood through these narrowed areas. This is akin to a clogged pipe in your house. If the pipe contains only a small amount of debris, the flow through the pipe will not be altered. Nothing will flow through the pipe, however, if it is clogged with a substantial amount of debris.

The problem with clogged arteries is that if there is diminished blood flow below the blockage (or no blood flow), oxygen and nutrients cannot be delivered to the tissues that are normally nourished by these vessels, causing the tissues to be significantly injured and die. Sometimes arteries become blocked gradually, but this can also occur quite suddenly, such as when a piece of debris breaks off and clogs a smaller blood vessel in another part of the body.

As mentioned earlier, multiple blood vessels can be affected by peripheral vascular disease. Typically, blood vessels in the legs are more affected than those in the arms. The same process that clogs arteries in the legs is also responsible for clogging arteries in the heart and brain, causing a heart attack or a stroke, respectively.

Symptoms of Peripheral Vascular Disease

PVD often causes pain in the legs that is made worse with walking, and relieved by rest. This is known as *intermittent claudication,* and may include feelings of heaviness, aching, or cramps in the calves. This pain occurs because the muscles that are used for walking are not getting enough oxygen and nutrients. Additionally, waste products are not being removed in a timely fashion.

If pain is also present at rest, a more severe clogging of the arteries in the legs is often the cause. This requires the attention of a physician.

Appearance of the Foot in Peripheral Vascular Disease

The foot may be shiny and pale, with little hair and a weak pulse. The color of the foot is important, because if it is blue, the blood supply to the foot may not be adequate. This is considered an emergency and, if not addressed immediately, may result in the loss of the limb.

Alternatively, the foot may be red when the feet are planted on the floor, but the redness goes away when the feet are elevated. This is known as *dependent rubor.*

The presence of an infection in the foot is suggested if the foot is warm, painful, and red. A discharge may or may not be present, and there may be fever and chills.

At times, a hole known as an *ulcer* or *ulceration* may develop in the foot. This means that the tissues of the foot have been injured and died. The tissues involved may be skin, muscle, or bone, depending on the depth of the ulcer.

Gangrene is a blackened color of the skin that indicates death of tissues.

Risk Factors for Peripheral Vascular Disease

The risk factors for PVD include diabetes, high blood pressure, high cholesterol, and smoking. In order to minimize your risks of developing PVD, check your blood pressure, sugar level, and cholesterol regularly, and adopt the appropriate lifestyle changes. If you are a smoker, STOP!

Your doctor will let you know if you also need to take any medications to bring these conditions under better control.

Diagnosis of Peripheral Vascular Disease

There are several ways that your doctor can assess the blood flow in your legs. Some of these tests are performed on the surface of the leg, and are considered *noninvasive.* Others require the insertion of various tubes and dyes. These procedures are considered *invasive.*

Noninvasive tests often include the use of blood pressure cuffs and a stethoscope to determine the blood flow in a limb. Ultrasound has also been used to visualize as well as approximate the amount of blockage that is present.

Invasive tests such as *angiography* are very useful in providing a detailed "picture" of the blood vessels in your leg. This procedure involves the injection of a dye into your blood stream, which can pose some health risks. Your doctor can describe these risks in detail.

The Treatment of Peripheral Vascular Disease

Depending on the severity of your PVD, the surgeon can attempt to open a clogged blood vessel or bypass it altogether. The bypass is accomplished by attaching a healthy donor blood vessel from another part of the body above and below the diseased blood vessel.

KEY POINTS

1. Peripheral vascular disease leads to a narrowing of blood vessels, which, in turn, cannot supply an adequate amount of blood to the tissues. As a consequence, the tissues do not get an adequate supply of nutrients and oxygen.

2. Common symptoms of PVD include heaviness, cramps, and aching sensations in the leg muscles. The feet may appear red or pale, and be cold. Pulses may also be faint or absent.

3. Risk factors for developing PVD include diabetes, high blood pressure, high cholesterol, and smoking.

4. It is very *important* to stop smoking if you are an active smoker.

5. The treatment of PVD includes controlling diabetes and high blood pressure, and reducing cholesterol. Medications and various types of surgeries may also be recommended.

CHAPTER 3

Prevention of Additional Amputations

This chapter is devoted to helping you avoid further amputation by taking care of your remaining limb, if you are deemed to be at high risk.

Your feet can withstand a great deal of pressure from everyday use, but they start to show wear and tear as you get older. This can be compounded by pain in other joints; for example, arthritis of the knee or hip.

Some common abnormalities of the toes include hammer toes, claw toes, or bunions. These abnormalities may lead to an abnormal pattern of walking, which puts pressure on certain aspects of the foot as opposed to others. These areas may develop more wear and tear than other parts of the foot.

The shoes that you wear on a daily basis may be too narrow in some areas, or may not give enough support to areas that need it the most (as in fallen arches).

Two of the most important risk factors for skin breaks in the feet are decreased sensation and decreased circulation. If you have poor sensation, you may not be aware of it when you step on a sharp object. You may also underestimate the severity of the problem because you do not feel the pain.

The following additional guidelines are adapted from some very good sources (1–3):

HOW TO INSPECT YOUR FEET

Inspect your feet daily. Check for any cracks, holes, calluses, or areas of redness or swelling. A *callus* is a hardening of the skin that is typically present over a bony prominence, such as the ball of the foot. It indicates an area of abnormal pressure on your foot. The callus may have a small opening leading to deeper layers of tissue, which can be a source of infection. Do not try to shave a callus down by yourself, because you may cause injury and possibly infection. Your foot doctor should treat a callus.

Areas of redness or swelling may indicate a possible site of infection, and should be monitored by your doctor closely. Ulcerations commonly occur on the ball of the foot, so it may be difficult for you to see them. Place a small mirror on the floor to inspect this area, or have a friend or family member examine the bottom of your feet once a day.

HOW TO WASH YOUR FEET

Use a soft cloth, warm water, and soap to wash your feet. Do not scrub the feet because it may irritate the skin. Check the water temperature with your elbow to make sure that it is not too hot. Your hands or feet may not be sensitive enough to test the temperature of the water. Dry the feet well, especially between the toes. Do not rub aggressively with a towel because this can also irritate the skin. Apply lotion after you have finished washing, but not between the toes. This will keep your skin moist and prevent cracks.

YOUR FEET AND SHARP OBJECTS

Do not use sharp objects on your feet, including nail files, scissors, or knives. These instruments can cause breaks in the skin, leading to infection. It is best to let a podiatrist take care of your feet.

SHOES AND SOCKS

It is a good policy not to walk barefoot on any surface. This is especially important at the beach or pool.

Wear cotton socks because they will absorb moisture and prevent damage to the skin. Socks should be loosely fitted so as not to cause an area of constriction.

Shoes should be comfortable and provide good support. They should not be constricting. Avoid open-toed, tight, pointed, or flat sandal-type shoes with no support, because they can be a source of injury. There should be adequate space for all the toes to move freely inside the shoe. Ideally, there should be about one-half of an inch between the toes and the front of the shoe when standing.

Your shoes should be made of a soft leather or canvas material that will absorb perspiration. They should have a wide and high toe box, and Velcro straps rather than laces, because laces are more difficult to tie if you have arthritis in your hands.

You may need an arch support or shoe modification if you have fallen arches or other foot problems. See a foot specialist before placing any inserts in your shoe. The wrong insert may cause areas of abnormal pressure and increase the risk of forming an ulceration. Make sure there are no sharp objects (such as nails or staples) inside your shoes before putting them on. Also, avoid using sharp objects to assist you in putting on your shoes.

KEY POINTS

1.   Inspect your feet daily—especially the bottoms.

2.   Do not walk barefoot, especially on rough, hot terrain (such as the beach).

3.   Avoid using sharp objects on your feet and see a podiatrist regularly.

4.   Invest in a good pair of shoes with a wide and high toe box.

5.   Keep your feet dry and wear cotton socks.

CHAPTER 4

Amputation Surgery

The decision to amputate a limb, or part of a limb, is not an easy one. It is typically made when the surgeon feels either that there is no way to preserve an adequate blood supply to the leg, or there is a significant life-threatening risk if amputation is *not* performed.

Once the decision to amputate is made, the *level* of amputation needs to be determined. The surgeon has various options, including amputating at the level of the toes, the forefoot, the ankle, below the knee, at the knee, above the knee, at the hip, or at the pelvis. This decision depends on how adequate the blood flow is to the remaining parts of the limb. Healing will be more successful after surgery if there is a good blood supply to the residual limb.

If the reason for the amputation is cancer in the limb, the surgeon must make sure that all of the cancer is removed. This will determine the level of the amputation.

When planning an amputation surgery, the surgeon will try not to amputate above-the-knee unless it is absolutely necessary, because it is easier to walk with a below-the-knee artificial limb (known as a *BK* or *transtibial prosthesis*) than an above the knee artifical limb (known as an *AK* or *transfemoral prosthesis*).

PARTIAL FOOT AMPUTATION

A foot can be amputated at the level of the toes, forefoot, or hind foot. A *forefoot (trans-metatarsal) amputation* is performed by making the cut just behind the ball of the foot. The tendons are allowed to retract into the remaining part of the foot. The longer, fleshier, bottom part of the foot is then attached to the shorter top of the foot.

ANKLE LEVEL AMPUTATION

A *Syme amputation* is performed at the level of the ankle. The remaining part of the heel is attached directly to the long bone of the calf (the *tibia*). The advantage of this type of amputation is that you can walk directly on the remaining limb once a socket and foot component is attached. It is therefore quite functional. The disadvantages are that it is not very cosmetic, and you may be limited in your choice of prosthetic feet.

BELOW-THE-KNEE AMPUTATION

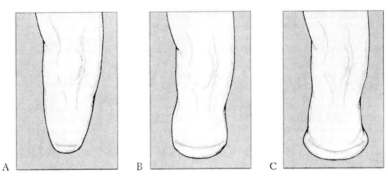

Figure 4-1 Residual limb shapes: A. conical; B. cylindrical; C. bulbous. (From R. Seymour, Prosthetics and Orthotics. Baltimore: Lippincott Williams & Wilkins, 2002. Reprinted by permission of the publisher.)

The *below-the-knee amputation (BKA)* is typically performed about 6 inches below the knee. A longer muscle flap made up of the thick muscles of the back of the calf is attached to the remaining part of the tibia or to a shorter muscle flap that makes up the front of the calf.

This soft tissue is important because it provides padding for the remaining part of the limb at the site where it attaches to the prosthesis. The remaining part of the limb is known as the *residual limb* or *stump.* It can have different shapes, but it is somewhat bulbous initially post-surgery because of swelling. In time, it may come to resemble a cylinder or a cone (Figure 4-1).

The length of the residual limb is very important. If it is too short or too long, it may be difficult to fit it with a prosthesis.

KNEE DISARTICULATION

Knee disarticulation surgery is a relatively rare type of amputation surgery in which the amputation is made directly through the knee itself. Douglas Smith, M.D., a noted expert in amputee surgery and care, has written about the advantages and disadvantages of this type of amputation (4).

Following a knee disarticulation amputation, the thigh bone and muscles remain intact and have a fairly well preserved appearance and strength, compared to an above-the-knee amputation. It may also be possible to bear more of the weight of the directly on the residual limb. It may also be more easy to put on and take off a prosthesis with a knee disarticulation amputation than with an above the knee amputation.

This type of amputation surgery can be especially useful for children who need a higher level of amputation, because the growth plates are preserved. This is important because it means that the femur in the affected leg will be the same size as the femur in the unaffected leg when the child reaches adulthood.

There are two main disadvantages to the knee disarticulation amputation. First, there is a loss of knee power, which can make it difficult to stand up from a seated position. Secondly, the residual limb may have a more bulbous appearance, which can make it less cosmetically appealing. The bulbous appearance does make it easier, however, to suspend a prosthesis from the residual limb.

ABOVE-THE-KNEE AMPUTATION

The *above-the-knee amputation (AKA)* is made through the thigh bone *(femur)* and thigh muscles. This is a fairly common site of amputation, although the trend in recent years has been more toward below the knee amputations.

Once the amputation is made, the remaining thigh muscles are attached to the remaining part of the femur. Ideally, the length of the remaining part of the limb is approximately 7 to 8 inches from the groin.

Once the muscles are cut, they will no longer function as well as they did prior to the amputation. They will be weaker, and have a tendency to pull the hip forward *(flexed)* and to the outside *(abducted)* . This may cause some irritation to the residual limb inside the prosthetic socket.

Douglas Smith has outlined several challenges faced by transfemoral amputees (5). Many of these are related to the loss of the knee. There is an increase in the energy required for ambulation with an AKA, as compared to a BKA. There may also be difficulties with balance, near-falls and falls, walking up and down stairs, and getting up and sitting down from a seated position.

HIP DISARTICULATION

Hip disarticulation surgery is reserved for people with cancer involving the thigh or higher, or for people with severe trauma of the leg. This amputation is performed very close to the hip socket, leaving the hip socket intact. Muscles from the buttocks are sewn to the remaining muscles of the inner thigh. This gives padding to the area that will be used to cushion the prosthesis, and also provides a more cosmetic look.

KEY POINTS

1. One of the most important decisions that a surgeon must make is the level at which to amputate. The site must have healthy tissue and good blood supply for adequate healing.

2. If at all possible, the knee should be spared, because it is more energy efficient and less difficult to walk with a below-the-knee amputation than an above-the-knee amputation.

CHAPTER 5

The Early Post-Surgical Period of Recovery

The early post-surgical period is the period of time between the surgery and transfer to a rehabilitation unit. This is approximately 1 to 3 weeks, barring any unexpected complications.

Up until now, the idea that you might need an amputation was just that—an idea. Now it has become a reality. Besides the immediate medical and surgical issues that need monitoring, your emotions will probably be somewhat unsettled. Feelings of loss, inadequacy, anger, and depression, as well as concerns about the future will occupy your thoughts.

You need support after your surgery! It can be helpful to talk to someone who is already living with an amputation. They will be able to give you information, strength, and advice. The rehabilitation department of your medical center can put you in contact with a representative from a local amputee support group. Another source of information may be a local veterans group.

COMMON PROBLEMS IMMEDIATELY AFTER SURGERY

The day-to-day issues you will confront are postoperative pain, wound healing, swelling of the residual limb (also known as *edema*), stiffness, and loss of motion in the residual limb.

You may experience pain for a variety of reasons, including pain in the residual limb from the surgery itself. Pain can also be caused by a nerve being trapped in scar tissue at the surgical site (this is often called a *neuroma*). *Phantom pain* is felt where the severed part of the limb used to be. This will be discussed in greater detail in Chapter 10.

The management of pain during the early post-surgical period typically involves the use of narcotic medications, such as oxycodone or morphine, which are taken at regular intervals. They may also be prescribed on a *per required need (PRN)* basis for breakthrough pain. Sometimes the surgeon or pain management physician will prescribe a *patient-controlled analgesia (PCA)* pump for several days post-surgery.

It is important to let your doctor, nurse, and therapist know if the medication prescribed is *not* adequately controlling your pain. Inadequately controlled pain can prevent you from fully participating in your therapy program. Ideally, you should ask for pain medication approximately 30 minutes before the start of your physical therapy sessions.

THE APPEARANCE OF THE RESIDUAL LIMB

The residual limb itself will be swollen and have a bulbous or flabby appearance after the surgery. There will also be stitches or staples in place. You will have the opportunity to look at the residual limb whenever the doctors or nurses inspect the wound. Take this opportunity to look at the residual limb, and also to touch it if your doctors allow it. This may be difficult to do, but the sooner that you re-establish the connection with your body, the better off you will be. Try to put a positive spin on the situation by realizing that the diseased part of your body was removed in order to save your life!

POSITIONING THE LIMB IN BED OR IN A WHEELCHAIR

Your natural tendency will be to keep the residual limb in positions that involve the least amount of pain, but these positions often promote stiffness and tightness in the hip and knee joints of the residual limb. The joints can "freeze" into a contracture, and you do not want to get a contracture! A contracture can interfere with the proper fitting of an artificial limb. It can also prolong your rehabilitation and make it difficult for you to walk with a prosthesis.

It is much better to prevent a contracture from developing than to treat one once it has developed. Some common tips for preventing contractures following BKA and AKA include:

Below-the-knee amputee

- Do not place a pillow under your knee.

- Do not dangle the residual limb when sitting on the side of your bed or in a chair or wheelchair.

- Keep the residual limb elevated on a well-padded board when sitting in a wheelchair.

- Avoid propping the residual limb on the sharp edges of chairs and other potentially sharp objects.

Above-the-knee amputee

- Do not sit in bed for prolonged periods of time. This can lead to contractures at your hips.

- Try to lie flat on your stomach for 15 to 20 minutes several times every day, if not medically contraindicated. This can help to prevent hip contractures from developing.

PHYSICAL AND OCCUPATIONAL THERAPY

Your doctor will determine when you are medically stable enough to begin therapy. This usually occurs a few days after the surgery. Your physical therapist and/or an occupational therapist will work with you toward several goals during the early post-surgical period.

Prevention of Contractures

Your therapist will work to prevent contractures from developing, or treat them if they have already formed. This is accomplished by moving the limb joints back and forth. This is especially important for the knee and hip on the affected side, but the remaining limbs also need to be exercised. You should get into the habit of moving the residual limb. The rationale is simple—the more you move the limb, the less likely that it will stiffen and freeze into a contracture.

Generalized Strengthening Program

You will need to strengthen the muscles in your arms, unaffected leg, and residual limb. You can lose a great deal of strength by staying in bed for a long period of time. This lost strength will make it more difficult for you to perform everyday activities when you go home. The exercises that the therapist recommends will focus on the muscle groups in your arms and legs that are important for walking and performing everyday activities, such as dressing, grooming, and hygiene.

You will need to work on getting up out of bed, transferring to a chair, and—when you are ready—hopping on your good leg with the help of a walker and a therapist.

Reduce Swelling of the Residual Limb

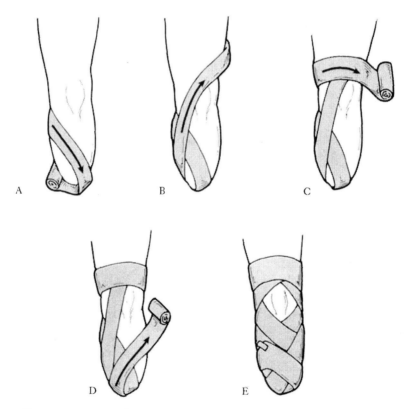

Figure 5-1 Figure-8 wrap or the transtibial amputation. (From R. Seymour, Prosthetics and Orthotics. Baltimore: Lippincott Williams & Wilkins, 2002. Reprinted by permission of the publisher.)

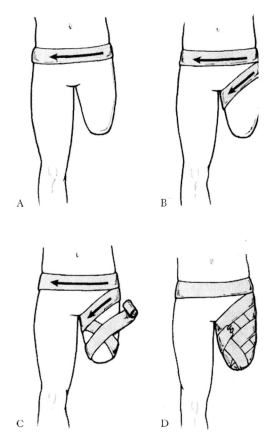

Figure 5-2 Transfemoral wrap. (From R. Seymour, Prosthetics and Orthotics. Baltimore: Lippincott Williams & Wilkins, 2002. Reprinted by permission of the publisher.)

The therapist will begin to work with you on various techniques to "shape" the residual limb. As mentioned earlier, your residual limb will be swollen immediately after surgery. In time, the swelling will decrease, but the sooner it decreases, the better. You will have less pain, better healing, and be fitted with a prosthesis sooner.

The therapist will wrap the residual limb with elastic bandages to reduce the swelling. She will also begin to teach you how to wrap it yourself. Become an active participant in your care by wrapping your residual limb as often as you can. Some common wrapping techniques are shown in Figures 5-1 and 5-2.

There are advantages and disadvantages in using an elastic bandage to reduce swelling. The main advantage is that you will learn self-care early in rehabilitation. It can also be useful in decreasing the swelling when other interventions are not possible. Bandages are typically applied several times every day. If you feel that the bandage is too tight, let the nurse, therapist, or doctor know so that it can be rewrapped.

There are two main disadvantages in using an elastic bandage. First, the tightness may not be evenly distributed along the entire residual limb, so that some areas may be tighter than others. Second, elastic bandages become loose quickly, causing them to lose their effectiveness. The bandage should be rewrapped several times every day.

Two other devices used to reduce swelling are the *shrinker* and the *immediate postoperative prosthesis (IPOP).* The shrinker is an elastic sock that is rolled onto the residual limb once the wound from the surgery is healed and the stitches or surgical staples are removed (Figure 5-3). It is typically worn most of the day, but your therapist or doctor can let you know the right amount of time for you.

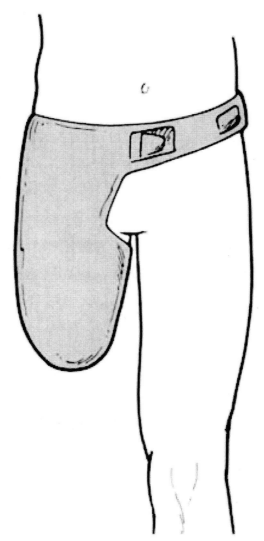

Figure 5-3 A shrinker may be used instead of elastic wraps. (From R. Seymour, Prosthetics and Orthotics.

Baltimore: Lippincott Williams & Wilkins, 2002.
Reprinted by permission of the publisher.)

You will continue to need the shrinker, even after you receive a prosthesis, as a way to keep swelling at a minimum. This is important because a swollen residual limb will make it more difficult to wear a prosthesis. A shrinker can be used to reduce swelling while you are waiting for repairs to be made to the prosthesis and it is not available for use, or if you have a medical condition that makes the limb swell periodically. The IPOP is a rigid cast that is applied to the residual limb immediately after surgery. It is similar to the type of cast that is used to immobilize a broken limb, but in this case it is used to minimize swelling. It also protects the residual limb from injury. The cast is typically made of plaster of paris or fiberglass. John Rhinestein, C.P. has written about the advantages and disadvantages of the IPOP (6):

- Reduces swelling and pain

- Provides protection to the residual limb when it is most vulnerable

- Prevents joint contractures

- Helps with transfers

The main drawback of IPOP is the potential for injury to the residual limb while it is being worn. The *removable rigid dressing* is an alternative to the IPOP. This is also a cast that is applied after surgery, but it can be removed for inspection. It is typically changed once it becomes loose. If your doctor provides you with this type of dressing, you should avoid using any sharp objects to scratch inside it because this may injure the skin. (Figure 5-4)

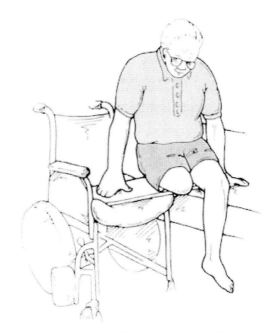

Figure 5-4 Use of a transfer board. (From R. Seymour, Prosthetics and Orthotics. Baltimore: Lippincott Williams & Wilkins, 2002. Reprinted by permission of the publisher.)

Training in Activities of Daily Living

The therapist will show you how to groom, bathe, and dress yourself to prepare you for your return home. Safe transfers from different surfaces, such as from a wheelchair to a bed or mat, are also emphasized. This often includes the use of a transfer board (Figure 5-4).

WOUND HEALING

Wound healing is of paramount importance. The wound is held together by staples or sutures, which allow the tissues and muscles to heal properly. They typically stay in place for 2 to 4 weeks, and are removed when the physician feels that adequate healing of the tissues has occurred.

Several factors are necessary for wound healing. It is important to maximize nutrition, keep sugar levels under control, maintain an adequate blood count, and treat infections quickly in order to give the residual limb the optimal chance of healing. Negative factors for healing include poor nutrition, inadequate blood supply, infection, low red blood cell count *(anemia)*, and diabetes. Signs of infection include redness at the wound line (also known as the *incision line*), fever, warmth, drainage, and/or a bad odor coming from the residual limb. Infections can occur superficially on the skin, in deeper tissues, or in the remaining bones. The type of antibiotic chosen depends on the site of the infection and the type of bacteria present at the wound site.

KEY POINTS

1. The most common concerns soon after amputation surgery are pain, problems with wound healing, infection, swelling of the residual limb, and contractures.

2. Care consists of pain management, optimizing nutrition, treatment of infections (if present), prevention of contractures, increasing overall body strength, and reducing swelling in the residual limb.

CHAPTER 6

The Rehabilitation Unit and the "Rehab" Team

Amputees are usually referred to a rehabilitation unit after surgery. These units are often part of the hospital where the surgery was performed. They may be a part of a nursing home or a large rehabilitation hospital. Most rehabilitation hospitals or units have a multidisciplinary team of specialists who work together to help the patient.

THE REHABILITATION TEAM

The "rehab" team typically includes a physician, rehabilitation nurse, physical therapist, occupational therapist, prosthetist, social worker, recreational therapist, and a psychologist.

Physiatrist

The physiatrist is a physician who has spent 4 years after medical school specializing in the rehabilitation of patients with various impairments and disabilities. His role is to coordinate all aspects of your care: medical, surgical, rehabilitation, and prosthetic. He will hold regular meetings with therapists and prosthetists to discuss your progress. He will also write the prescription for your prosthesis.

Physical Therapist

This health care professional will work with you to improve your lower body strength and transfer skills, and reduce the swelling in your residual limb. She will also help you with prosthetic training once the prosthesis is delivered. Physical therapists are also knowledgeable about various modalities, such as ice, heat, ultrasound, and electrical stimulation. Physical therapy assistants often help the physical therapist.

Occupational Therapist

This health care professional will teach you how to perform the activities of daily living, such as dressing, bathing, and grooming. He is also an expert on various adaptive devices that make it easier to perform these activities. The occupational therapist often "co-treats" with a physical therapist.

Prosthetist

The prosthetist is the member of the rehab team who is responsible for fabricating the prosthesis. She will assist the physiatrist and the physical therapist in identifying the best prosthetic components to achieve your ambulation goals. A good working relationship with your prosthetist is very important. This relationship may last for many years, as your prosthetic needs and prosthetic technology change.

Rehabilitation Nurse

The rehabilitation nurse is experienced in the care of patients with various impairments and disabilities. He is knowledgeable about medications and bowel, bladder, skin, and wound care. A credentialing process certifies a nurse with experience or training as a rehabilitation nurse.

Social Worker

The social worker specializes in the understanding of health benefits and patient rights. She can help you navigate through the complex financial and health care insurance issues. Social workers are often very good at counseling and teaching coping skills.

Recreation Therapist

The recreation therapist will provide different diversions while you are on the rehab unit. He is knowledgeable about leisure and recreational activities, and incorporates them into the rehabilitation process. He can also be a resource for the community leisure activities that are accessible for individuals with physical disabilities.

Psychologist

The psychologist will help you adjust to life without a limb. She also teaches coping skills and screens for depression or other psychological illnesses that can affect rehabilitation.

COORDINATION OF CARE ON THE REHAB UNIT

Each team member will perform an individual assessment of your needs, and then meet with the rest of the rehab team to discuss your particular strengths and weaknesses. Do not be surprised if more than one person asks you how many steps you have at the entrance of your home or how you managed your own cooking before the surgery. These are standard questions to assess your lifestyle prior to the surgery and identify your needs upon your return home.

Once this information is collected, a *team meeting* will be held by everyone involved in your care. You and your spouse or significant other will need to attend this meeting because it is a forum at which you can ask the questions that are important to you.

At the meeting, an initial plan of care will be developed to address any barriers that prevent you from returning home. Goals and an estimated length of stay on the rehab unit will be set. A typical length of stay on a rehab unit for pre-prosthetic training is 2 to 4 weeks.

During your stay on the rehabilitation unit, team meetings will be held weekly or every 2 weeks. Everyone involved in your care will provide an update on your progress during these meetings. As each goal is met, a new one may be added. Eventually, the team will decide that you are ready to return to your home and the community, and a discharge date will be set.

THE REHABILITATION PROGRAM

Your program on the rehabilitation unit will be comparable to the therapy that you received immediately after your surgery, but it will last for several hours each day and be more intense. The goals will be more or less the same:

- Complete wound healing

- Strengthen muscles in all the limbs, including the remaining muscles of the amputated limb

- Reduce swelling in the residual limb

- Maximize your functional level for the activities of daily living

A physician will monitor your medical condition, calling medical and surgical consultations as needed. The physician and his staff will also stay in contact with your family and insurance company to update them on your progress.

SURGICAL WOUND HEALING

You cannot be fitted with a temporary prosthesis until the residual limb is completely healed. The stress of wearing a hard plastic shell around fragile skin can lead to breakdown of the wound and possibly infection. This breakdown can cause further complications that may prolong your hospitalization.

If your wound has not completely healed, but you have completed your rehab goals with respect to strength training and functional activities, your physician may recommend that you be discharged to a nursing home or sent home with visiting nurse services until the wound heals.

Once the wound is completely healed, you can be readmitted to the rehab unit for prosthetic training. You can also receive this training in the nursing home or be fitted with a prosthesis as an outpatient and learn how to walk with it in an outpatient therapy clinic.

These decisions often depend on your level of support at home, your ability to travel for outpatient services, or the proximity of your family or caretakers to the rehabilitation facility. Your insurance may also dictate the location and terms of your rehabilitation.

KEY POINTS

1. The best way to care for someone who has sustained an amputation is with the team approach. Given the complexity of the issues involved, a stay in a rehabilitation unit is strongly advised.

2. A team of rehab professionals meets regularly on the rehabilitation unit to discuss the progress and problems encountered by the amputee. This team typically consists of a physician, physical therapist, occupational therapist, recreational therapist, social worker, psychologist, rehabilitation nurse, and prosthetist.

CHAPTER 7

The Prosthesis

Not everyone who has a limb amputated needs or wants a prosthesis. You may decide that your lifestyle is sufficiently sedentary, and you do not need a prosthesis. There is a lot to learn when it comes to using a prosthesis. It will be one less headache if you can manage to have an independent lifestyle without one!

In some circumstances, your doctor may advise you not to get a prosthesis. For example, it may be difficult for you to learn to walk safely with one if you have a learning impairment. It can also be dangerous for you to use a prosthesis if you have a severe balance deficit and fall a great deal. If your physician and therapist think that you can learn to use a prosthesis, you owe it to yourself to try. You have to be motivated, willing to learn, and work hard. You will have overcome one of your life's greatest challenges if you are able to master using a prosthesis!

THE TIMING OF PROSTHESIS FITTING

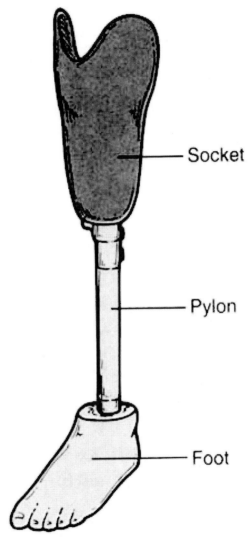

Figure 7-1 Adjustable prosthesis used in early gait training under the supervision of a physical therapist. (Adapted from a drawing by Campbell Childs Inc.; from R. Seymour, Prosthetics and Orthotics. Baltimore: Lippincott Williams & Wilkins, 2002. Reprinted by permission of the publisher.)

The two main criteria for determining the timing of fitting a prosthesis are (1) the residual limb is completely healed, and (2) you have the stamina and body strength necessary to hop 50 to 100 feet using a walker. If you meet these criteria and there are no medical contraindications, there is a very good chance that you will be fitted with your first prosthesis (also known as a *temporary prosthesis*) while on the rehabilitation unit (Figure 7-1).

The temporary prosthesis is a basic device that is used to teach you how to walk and perform daily functions safely with an artificial limb. It has the following components:

- Suspension system—needed to suspend the prosthesis from the body

- Socket—the shell that is in immediate contact with the residual limb

- Shank—the metal piece that connects the socket or prosthetic knee to the foot

- Knee component (for an above the knee prosthesis)

- Prosthetic foot

The components used to fabricate the prosthesis are chosen with safety and stability in mind. These components will be discussed later in greater detail.

The socket is fabricated by the prosthetist, who will wrap your residual limb with sheets of plaster of paris to create a *negative mold.* The negative mold is then filled with plaster to create a *positive mold.* Next, the socket is fabricated as a shell based on the positive mold. (This is a painless process.)

The other components are attached to the socket to complete the temporary prosthesis. The prosthetist typically completes the temporary prosthesis within 1 to 4 weeks.

FACTORS INVOLVED IN PRESCRIBING A PROSTHESIS

Your prosthesis will be custom-made to your specifications from carefully selected components based on your needs and medical condition. A great deal of thought and planning go into making it. Many factors must be considered when prescribing a prosthesis for the lower limb. The team of specialists involved in your care will consider your medical condition, lifestyle, and wishes. The two worst things that could happen are: (1) you will be given an inadequate prosthesis and never use it, or (2) you receive an inadequate prosthesis that puts you at risk for falling and injuring yourself.

Your physician will ask about your lifestyle before the surgery. Were you active before the amputation or were you a limited ambulator? Did you use any assistive devices for walking?

It is also important to know about your living arrangements. Do you live alone or with a family member or friend? Do you live in an apartment or a house? Are there stairs where you live? It is also important to know how you carried out the activities of daily living, such as bathing, grooming, dressing, shopping, and driving, prior to the surgery. Were you able to perform these activities on your own, or did you need assistance?

Your physician will also rely on input from the therapists currently treating you. He will want to know if you are alert, motivated, and able to learn how to safely put on a prosthesis and ambulate with it.

The physician's examination typically focuses on vision, hand and upper body strength, and range of motion in the limbs. Fitting a prosthesis is more difficult if there is a contracture. The physician will pay careful attention to the length, circumference, and shape of your residual limb. Length is especially important. If the residual limb is too short or too long, it may cause problems with fitting the prosthesis. The surgery site should be clean, dry, and intact. There should be no evidence of breaks in the skin or any signs of infection. Although the surgery site on the residual limb may be somewhat tender to touch, any unusually tender areas will need to be noted so that they can be given extra protection.

The skin should be loosely attached to the underlying tissues at the surgery site. The skin may be at risk for future breaks if it is too tightly attached to the underlying bone.

The presence of swelling (edema) is also important. Although edema is quite common after amputation surgery, there are also medical conditions that cause *fluctuating edema,* a condition in which the swelling varies from day to day. For example, patients on *hemodialysis* may have this problem. Edema affects the decision as to when to fit the prosthesis.

TEMPORARY AND PERMANENT PROSTHESES

A new prosthesis is like a new shoe. It needs to be broken in gradually. The skin can become irritated or torn if you wear it too long and the fit is not good. Initially, you should limit wearing the temporary prosthesis to about 15 minutes during your therapy sessions on the rehab unit. You can gradually increase the wearing time to 1 to 2 hours per day if it is tolerated well. You should always check your skin after wearing your prosthesis.

You will use the temporary prosthesis primarily for learning how to stand, walk, and turn safely. You will use it on different surfaces, stairs, and getting in and out of a car.

The temporary prosthesis is usually worn for a period of 6 to 12 months. During this time, the shape of the residual limb will mature, and swelling will be reduced to a minimum. Your prosthetist will be able to make adjustments to the prosthesis to accommodate your needs and walking style. Your input is very important.

A common question amputees ask is: "How will I know when I am ready for a permanent prosthesis?" The answer to this question depends on the changes in the size of the residual limb over time. Initially, it will be very swollen, but the swelling will decrease as you ambulate. As the swelling of the residual limb decreases, you will find that your residual limb comes into greater contact with the bottom of the socket, perhaps causing discomfort. You may feel that you are "pistoning" in and out of the socket.

You will typically wear one or more specially designed socks while using the temporary prosthesis. These socks vary in thickness, and are a barrier between your skin and the socket. The thickness of each sock is measured in *ply.* Typically, socks come in 1, 3, 5, and 6-ply thicknesses. Initially, you may need only one 5-ply sock, but you may eventually need to add two or more socks of varying thickness to accommodate the volume loss. Knowing when to add or subtract socks is often more of an art than an exact science. Your therapist or prosthetist can help you make this decision.

You may find that you need to add more and more socks to keep your residual limb from moving inside the socket. It is time to talk to your physician or prosthetist about a new socket or permanent prosthesis when you are wearing more than a total of 13 to 15 ply socks. (It is common to have one or sometimes more temporary sockets fabricated before the permanent one is made.)

COMPONENTS OF THE BKA PROSTHESIS

There are four main components of a BKA prosthesis:

Suspension

A suspension device attaches the prosthesis to the remaining portion of the limb or the waist. This device ensures that the prosthesis will not fall off the residual limb. The major advantage of having a good suspension system is that your prosthesis will fit better, and it will be easier to walk with it. There will also be less irritation to the skin or tears in the skin. There are several types of suspension systems:

SUPRACONDYLAR SUSPENSION. This type of suspension has extra material added to the sides of the socket that enables it to suspend itself from the ends of the femur (thigh bone). This bone has terminal ends known as *condyles,* hence the term supracondylar suspension. Often a strap above the kneecap supplements this type of suspension, especially in less active ambulators who need extra support (Figure 7-2). A similar type of suspension is the *supracondylar/suprapatellar,* in which extra material is added above the kneecap as well as to the sides of the socket. This is indicated if you have a short residual limb. The disadvantage of this type of suspension is that it can be more noticeable under clothing and may limit the range of motion of the knee during ambulation. (Figure 7-2)

ELASTIC SLEEVE. This type of suspension is basically a rubber sleeve that is attached to the socket and "rolled over" the upper part of the socket and onto the thigh. It is a very common type of suspension when used alone or as a secondary suspension for patients with suction suspension (see below). The disadvantages of this type of suspension include the retention of heat and moisture. It may also irritate the skin or cause allergic skin reactions. A certain amount of hand strength and dexterity is also required to put it on and take it off.

THIGH CORSET. This type of suspension has metal bars on the sides of the knee and a corset (leather cuff) with laces on the thigh. This is not a very common type of suspension because it is heavy, bulky, and requires good hand strength and dexterity. This type of suspension is indicated if you have a short residual limb and knee instability.

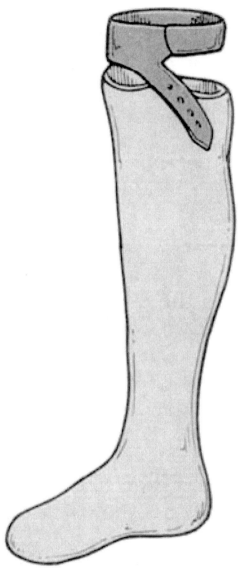

Figure 7-2 Supracondylar cuff suspension. (Adapted from Shurr, DG & Cook, TM. Prosthetics and Orthotics. Norwalk, CT: Appleton & Lange; from R. Seymour, Prosthetics and Orthotics. Baltimore: Lippincott Williams & Wilkins, 2002. Reprinted by permission of the publisher.)

PIN/SHUTTLE SYSTEM. This has become a very popular type of suspension. It consists of a sock made out of a gel-like material (silicone) that has a pin attached at the bottom. This pin "locks-in" to the bottom of the socket and suspends the prosthesis. The pin is unlocked by pressing a button on the socket. There are several advantages to this type of suspension—it is light, easy to roll on, and provides less friction to the skin. This last point is especially important if you have fragile skin that is close to the bone. The disadvantage of this type of suspension is that it places greater stress on painful arthritic hands and needs regular cleaning. Good hygiene is very important, and frequent washing of the residual limb and gel liner is essential.

SUCTION SUSPENSION. Suction suspension is based on the principle that by inserting the residual limb in a socket with a one-way air valve at the bottom, you push out all of the air in the socket as the residual limb is advanced inside. This creates a negative pressure or vacuum in the socket, thereby suspending the prosthesis. This is a very good type of suspension.

Suction suspension is indicated if you have a well-shaped residual limb that does not change very much in size. It is not indicated if your residual limb has a great deal of scarring or has a very fleshy, irregularly shaped appearance that changes in thickness on a daily basis. This may occur if you are on dialysis or have a heart problem that predisposes you to retain water. The reason for these contraindications is that, if present, it is difficult to maintain a good suction inside the socket. A suction suspension system requires greater than average hand strength and effort to put on and take off.

Socket

The socket is a plastic shell that fits over the residual limb and connects the prosthesis to the body. It is designed to apply pressure to the soft fleshy areas, such as muscles, and not to bony surfaces. These areas include the fleshy sides of the shin bone, the soft tendon area just below the kneecap, the back of the knee, the flares of the shin bone by the knee, and the bottom of the residual limb. The amount of force placed on the bottom of the residual limb should be kept to a minimum, however, because excessive pressure may lead to irritation and injury.

The socket is meant to maintain total contact with the residual limb, but because it is not a part of the residual limb, but merely an appendage, there will always be some slight movement of the limb within it.

Most sockets have a soft inner liner that provides extra padding and comfort to the residual limb (especially the bony areas). The liner is made of silicone or a light urethane material. Silicone gel is helpful in reducing friction between the socket and the skin.

Shank

The shank is the calf component of the prosthesis. It connects the socket to the foot. The shank may be in the shape of a tube *(endoskeletal)* or a shell *(exoskeletal)*. The tube type is lighter, and its alignment with the respect to the other components can be adjusted by the prosthetist.

The exoskeletal shank is very hardy and can withstand abuse. It is typically considered for people who will not be able to get to a prosthetist very often and need a shank that does not need much maintenance. The drawback is that it is very difficult to adjust once it is fabricated.

Prosthetic Feet

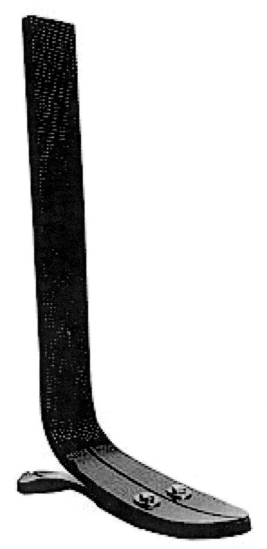

Figure 7-3 Flex foot. (Photo courtesy of Ossur.)

A great deal has been written about prosthetic feet. Many companies have devised different types of feet for different users. The goal is always the same: Create a foot that can duplicate the functions of the human foot—as much as possible—during stance and ambulation on different surfaces.

One of the most important things that you can tell your doctor and prosthetist is how you plan on using your prosthesis. Are you going to do most of your walking around your home? Do you plan on hiking or playing golf? They will prescribe an appropriate prosthetic foot depending on your answers.

If you are not going to do much walking outside of the home, your doctor may prescribe a *solid ankle cushioned heel (SACH) foot.* This is a very durable type of foot with a soft rubber heel. It is typically prescribed if you are a limited ambulator or if you are still learning how to use a prosthesis. It may also be recommended if you are not able to come in for regular follow-up visits to the prosthetist.

If you plan on walking outside the home on a regular basis, you may benefit from a more dynamic, "energy-storing foot" that gives you more "spring" when you walk. This tends to be more expensive than the SACH foot, but it may be better suited to your needs.

There are many different types of dynamic, energy-storing feet. They are based on the principle that energy is stored in the heel of the foot when the heel strikes the ground. That energy is used to give you a "spring" when your toes push off the ground (Figure 7-3).

The type of foot that is prescribed also depends on where you live. If you live in an area that is subject to harsh weather conditions, your prosthetist may recommend a foot that is simpler in design and more durable. This is because some of the components in the prosthetic foot may be damaged by excessive water, mud, or dust. Your insurance company may also place restrictions on the type of prosthetic components you are prescribed.

If you are an active person, you will probably walk on different surfaces every day. Prosthetic feet are meant to accommodate your walking style on both flat and uneven terrain using a hybrid design. They can be used for walking inside your home or while jogging or playing tennis.

Some types of feet can be adjusted by the wearer, depending on how they are going to be used. These include the Dynamic Response 2 Foot (manufactured by Endolite North

America, Centerville, OH), and the Masterstep Foot (manufactured by Cascade Orthopedic Supply, Chico, CA). Other types of feet have a shock-absorbing system built into a single combined foot and shank unit (Re-Flex VSP Standard, manufactured by Flex Foot Inc., Aliso Viejo, CA). Some types of feet are said to be waterproof (DynaSTEP foot, manufactured by DAW Industries, San Diego, CA).

The technology of prosthetic feet is constantly changing. Your prosthetist can keep you abreast of the latest designs and whether they are suitable for you.

COMPONENTS OF THE AKA PROSTHESIS

The AKA prosthesis has five components (Figure 7-4):

Suspension

The suspension devices for the AKA prosthesis are similar to those available for the BKA prosthesis. Their main function is to attach the prosthesis to the remaining portion of the limb or the waist. (Figure 7-4)

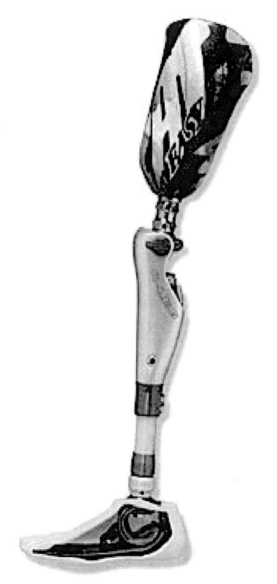

Figure 7-4 C-Leg. (Reprinted with permission from Otto Bock Orthopedic Industry Inc Minneapolis, MN).

SUCTION SUSPENSION. This type of suspension is also offered if you have an above-the-knee prosthesis. This is a very good type of suspension. It is indicated for an active person with good balance and strength. The suction suspension is applied in one of two ways. The first is by putting on a sock and then inserting the residual limb into the socket. The sock is then pulled out through a hole (also known as a *valve housing*) in the bottom of the socket. This hole also acts as a one-way air valve. The valve is screwed into the housing when the sock is pulled out. A negative pressure system is generated within the socket, which holds it in place (Figure 7-5).

Another way of applying suction suspension does not involve guide socks. You simply apply a powder to the residual limb and then insert the limb directly into the socket. As you advance the limb inside the socket, the air is expelled out through the hole with a one-way valve. This creates a negative pressure system that holds the limb in place. The suction suspension system can be supplemented by a waist belt if you are very active.

You need good hand strength to use a suction socket. You should also be free of any major heart problems, because the extra effort used in applying it can place a greater stress on your heart.

The same limitations noted for the below-the-knee suction system apply for the above the knee suction system. The limb should be of a

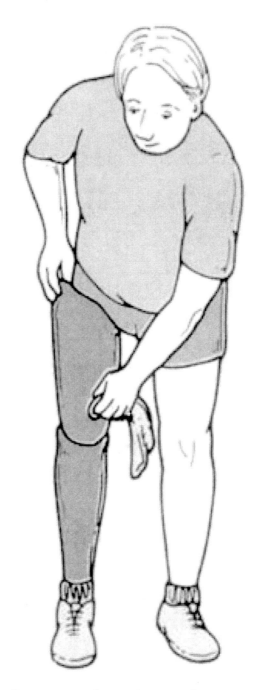

Figure 7-5 Application of traditional suction suspension. (From R. Seymour, Prosthetics and Orthotics. Baltimore: Lippincott Williams & Wilkins, 2002. Reprinted by permission of the publisher.)

stable volume and thickness, and have little scarring. Ideally, the thigh muscles should be firm (not flabby), because this may interfere with the creation of the negative pressure system. Given the greater effort involved in putting on the socket, your physician may recommend against it if you have a heart condition.

PIN/LOCK SYSTEMS. A silicone liner with a pin can also be used in the AKA prosthesis. It is worn between the residual limb and the socket. It has thicker padding at the bottom to provide extra cushioning for the thigh bone, and it is thinner at the top for comfort. There is a pin at the bottom of the gel liner, which attaches or "locks" into the bottom of the socket when the residual limb is placed inside. This type of suspension is recommended for the person who is sedentary and has fluctuation in the size of their residual limb.

Sometimes it is difficult to insert the pin into the lock because you cannot see the direction it is going inside the socket. A device known as the *locking lanyard* can be of help. This is a cord that is attached to the bottom of the liner, which then guides the residual limb and the liner pin into the lock. According to Jennifer Dowell, C.P.O., this can be very useful for

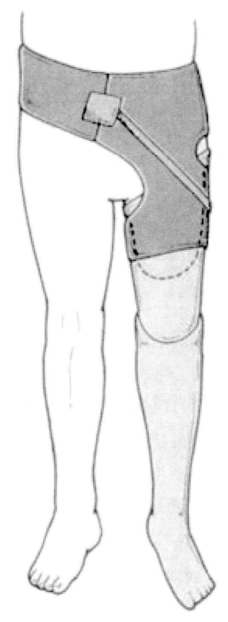

Figure 7-6 Total elastic suspension (TES). (From R. Seymour, Prosthetics and Orthotics. Baltimore: Lippincott Williams & Wilkins, 2002. Reprinted by permission of the publisher.)

above-the-knee amputees who are unstable when attempting to put on a prosthesis while in the upright position.

TOTAL ELASTIC SUSPENSION BELT (TES). This is a belt made of a soft plastic material known as *neoprene* (Figure 7-6). This type of suspension belt attaches to the socket and encircles your waist. It is held in place by a Velcro fastener. The advantage of this type of suspension is that is elastic, making it somewhat easier to put on.

The TES can serve as a secondary type of suspension for active amputees who have a prosthesis with suction suspension. This is a very good alternative if you cannot be fitted with a suction suspension. The disadvantage of the TES is that it retains heat and moisture and can become somewhat uncomfortable to wear. It may not last very long because it is made of elastic. (Figure 7-6)

SILESIAN BELT. This is a belt that attaches to the socket and encircles the waist at the level of the pelvis (Figure 7-7). It prevents the prosthesis from moving on the thigh or trunk if you have flabby skin. This type of belt is recommended if the total elastic suspension belt does not provide adequate suspension. This

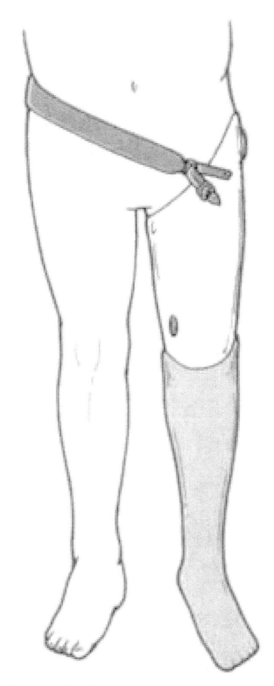

Figure 7-7 Silesian belt suspension. (From R. Seymour, Prosthetics and Orthotics. Baltimore: Lippincott Williams & Wilkins, 2002. Reprinted by permission of the publisher.)

is a good secondary suspension that can be used with a suction suspension system if you are active and athletic. This type of belt may irritate the areas where there are sensitive scars because of its close contact with the skin. It is contraindicated if you have significant problems with your hip on the amputated side. (Figure 7-7)

PELVIC BELT AND HIP JOINT. This type of suspension uses a metal or plastic joint to attach the socket to a belt made of leather (Figure 7-8), which encircles the waist. It is indicated for people who have short residual limbs and instability around the hip joint. There are many disadvantages to this type of suspension, limiting its use. It is heavy, bulky, and not very cosmetic. The leather belt can also get dirty from poor hygiene.

Socket

The AKA socket attaches to the residual limb in a manner similar to the BKA. The socket is the "link" between the residual limb and the prosthesis. Therefore, it is very important that there is a good fit. Two types of sockets are available: *quadrilateral* and *ischial containment.* These terms refer to the shape of the socket, and whether or not the *ischium bone* is inside

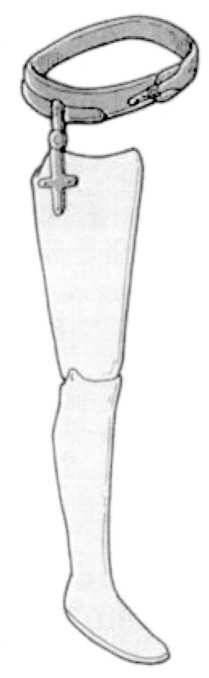

Figure 7-8 Pelvic band and hip joint suspension. (From R. Seymour, Prosthetics and Orthotics. Baltimore: Lippincott Williams & Wilkins, 2002. Reprinted by permission of the publisher.)

or outside of the socket when the prosthesis is being worn. The ischium bone is a part of the pelvis that is commonly felt when sitting on your buttocks. (Figure 7-8)

Ischial containment sockets are more commonly used because they are believed to give better control of the long bone of the femur and the ischium. They increase comfort and offer better control of the prosthesis during ambulation by providing a better fit. This type of socket is better suited for active ambulators. One disadvantage is that the prosthesis can rotate while sitting, causing the prosthetic foot to point inward.

In the past, the materials used to fabricate sockets were hard and rigid. Now there are new types of sockets that combine hard elements (applied where extra support is needed), with lighter materials to improve comfort and decrease weight.

Knee

Several types of knee units are available. Some are geared toward people with limited ambulation and emphasize safety and stability. This type includes the *manual locking knee.* Others provide a more natural and fluid movement;

for example, *hydraulic* and *fluid-controlled knees.*

John W. Michael is a leading prosthetist who has written and lectured a great deal on prostheses and prosthetic knees. In recent articles written in an orthopedic journals he wrote about the five basic types of prosthetic knees (7, 8):

- Single axis

- Weight-activated stance control

- Polycentric

- Manual-locking

- Fluid-controlled

The remainder of this chapter discusses some of John W. Michael's findings and recommendations, and relates the author's own experience as well.

In order to understand how the prosthetic knee works, you have to understand what your physical knee did for you. First, it provided you with stability every time you took a step by locking in place, so that your leg could support your body without buckling. Obviously, you would fall if it buckled. This locking was aided by the muscles in the front of your thigh known as the *quadriceps.*

Secondly, there was built-in resistance within the knee that you could use to vary the speed at which the knee bent. This was important in allowing you to walk at different speeds. This resistance was provided by internal structures within the knee as well as by the muscles around it. Your brain would instruct these muscles how hard and fast they should contract to produce the desired effect. Prosthetic knees attempt to duplicate one or both of these functions.

The *single axis knee* is also known as the *free-swinging knee.* It is less expensive and more durable and reliable. Its main disadvantage is that you can only walk at one speed when using it. You cannot vary your speed from slow to fast. Also, it does not offer much support, and you may buckle when walking. You need to have good thigh muscle strength to use this type of knee. It is not good for older, frail, limited ambulators because it can increase the risk of falling.

The *weight-activated stance control knee* has an internal brake that provides constant friction as you walk, decreasing the likelihood that your knee will buckle. This knee does not bend when your body weight is shifted above it, but rather bends once the weight is taken. It provides a considerable amount of stability when you need it the most. This type of knee is indicated if you are just learning how to walk with a prosthesis or if safety (from falling) is a major concern. There are two disadvantage to this type of knee: The brake can fail, and there is a limit to the amount of bending that can be done.

The *polycentric knee* has multiple centers of rotation. The center of the rotation changes as the knee bends. It has two important advantages: stability and an ability to bend with greater ease. This makes it easier to use when walking on different surfaces and at different speeds. It is commonly prescribed as a knee component for people who are just beginning to walk with a temporary prosthesis. It can also be used as a part of a permanent prosthesis if you require greater stability but are able to walk at different speeds. The author commonly uses this type of knee with his older patients.

The *manual-locking knee* is locked into position by manipulating a lever. Once locked, you will walk with a straight, stiff, "peg leg" type of gait. As a result, your ability to walk will not be smooth and efficient. There may also be a problem when you try to sit down, because you will have to manually unlock the knee to be able to bend it and then sit. This type of knee is not typically used, and has been described by John W. Michael as "a knee of last resort." Nevertheless, it is the most stable type of prosthetic knee, and can be beneficial if you have a significant balance problem or need to walk on uneven terrain.

The *fluid-controlled knee* has a chamber that is filled with air or oil. The materials in this chamber are not compressed very well, and offer resistance to the speed of the knee movements as you go from bent to straight. You will be able to walk at different speeds with a smoother more normal walking style when using this type of knee. John W. Michael thinks that this type of knee should be offered to amputees who can walk on different surfaces and at different speeds.

If you walk slowly and steadily, and do not vary your walking speed very much, this type of knee is not for you. Typically, this knee is more expensive and requires more maintenance than other types of prosthetic knees. The author recommends this type of knee for his patients who are active community ambulators and can walk at different speeds.

Some prosthetic knees have *combined* key elements of the polycentric knee, stance-control knee, and hydraulic knee to create a hybrid design that takes advantage of the best features of all of them (Figure 7-9).

The *C-leg* (manufactured by Otto Block Orthopedic Industry Inc.) has a built-in microprocessor that interprets information about the knee's position in space and speed of movement during walking in order to adjust the resistance within the knee (see Figure 7-4). This provides a smoother walk on varied surfaces and inclines, offering knee stability when required.

Shank and Foot

Both the shank and foot share the same characteristics and limitations as the BKA prosthesis. (Figure 7-9)

Special Components

John W. Michael has also written about special adaptive devices that can be of great help to the above-the-knee amputee. One such device is called a *locking transverse rotation unit.* This device is placed just above the prosthetic knee. When you are seated, you will be able to rotate the knee-shank-foot components more than 90 degrees. This can be of help if you want to get in and out of a seat in a narrow space with greater ease, such as the car or the seat in a movie theater (9).

KEY POINTS

1. The minimum criteria needed to be fitted with a prosthesis are: a healed residual limb, good balance, good strength, and endurance that enables you to hop with a walker for about 50 feet.

2. The temporary prosthesis is the first prosthesis you will receive. You will use it to learn how to walk with an artificial limb. Approximately 6 to 12 months after receiving the temporary prosthesis, you will be ready to be fitted with your permanent prosthesis.

3. A prosthesis is made up of several different components: suspension system, socket; shank, knee component, and a prosthetic foot.

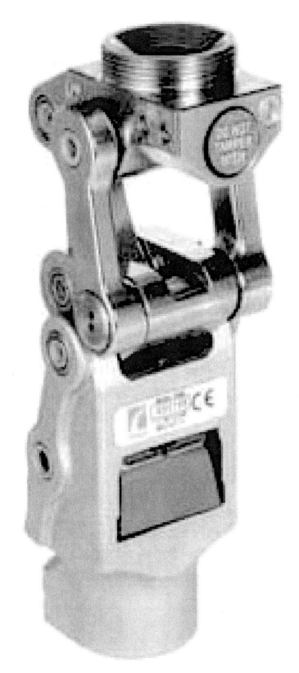

Figure 7-9 Total knee. (Photo courtesy of Ossur.)

4. Each component comes in several different styles, some of which are better for more active people, and some for more sedentary

ones. Your lifestyle and the rehab team will decide the choice of components. It is important that you give them as much information as you can regarding your lifestyle and needs.

CHAPTER 8

Walking with a Prosthesis

This chapter discusses two very important topics: (1) walking with a lower limb prosthesis, and (2) common abnormal walking patterns with a prosthesis and what can be done to correct them.

Learning to walk with a prosthesis is very individualized. You may learn quickly, or it may take you a while. The level of use may also vary—you may use it to walk around your home or you may run races.

The difference between walking with a prosthesis and the regular walking you have done all your life boils down to one thing—energy consumption! It takes more energy to walk wearing a prosthesis than it does to walk on two legs. BK amputees consume about 30 percent more energy, and AK amputees consume about 80 percent more energy walking than people without a lower limb amputation.

This does not necessarily mean that you will walk less, but rather that it will take you longer to cover the same distance. Of course, there is a great deal of variability between one person and another. A younger person with a below the knee amputation sustained in a traumatic event may be in better shape overall than an older, frail person with multiple medical problems. As a result, their walking speeds and the distances covered will probably differ.

FUNDAMENTALS OF WALKING AND ENERGY CONSUMPTION

In order to understand the process of walking with a prosthesis, you must understand the process of walking on two sound limbs. The first and foremost principle is that the body tries to conserve as much energy as possible during walking, because the body has a finite amount of energy available to carry out every-day activities. Energy is the end product of the food and water consumed daily. It is used to carry out all of the biological functions, including keeping the body moving. Energy is also used as a source of nourishment by your brain, which coordinates all the movements of the body.

Every activity that you perform during the day uses energy. Whether you are sitting comfort-ably in a chair reading this book, running to catch a bus, or playing with your children or grandchildren, everything has an energy cost to your body. Therefore, your body tries to be as efficient as possible, causing you to feel tired when your energy supply dwindles.

This is analogous to a car, which needs gasoline to make the engine run. A heavy car with many features is less energy efficient and uses more gasoline. A lighter car with an energy efficient design requires less gasoline. Engineers who design cars try to make them as energy efficient as possible in order to get the most energy from the least amount of gas.

The human musculoskeletal system is a marvelous piece of engineering. It is designed to keep the total number of muscles contracting at any given time to a minimum. This is important because the more muscles that work at the same time, the more energy is consumed and the least distance you can go before you get tired. For example, if you are standing in line at the supermarket, only a few of the muscles in your legs are contracting. This is primarily accomplished with the support of certain *ligaments* (nonmuscular structures), located in front of your hips and behind your knees. The muscles and ligaments work together to keep the legs locked in a straight position in order to hold the body upright. The major muscles that contract during standing are those in the front and back of the calves. The muscle group in the back of the calves is known as the *gastrocnemius.* The one in the front of the thigh is known as the *anterior tibialis.* They each contract for a short period of time. This enables you rock back and forth in place. When you stand on your toes, the gastrocnemius is contracting. When you stand on your heels, the anterior tibialis is contracting. An additional muscle group that is important for standing upright is the quadriceps. This muscle group keeps the knee straight by contracting.

Various muscle groups contract in a sequential fashion when needed for walking. Then they quickly stop contracting, giving them a chance to rest. This also keeps the energy cost down. The highest cost of energy during walking results from the contraction of the muscles that help stabilize the joints in one limb while the other limb is advancing forward.

There is an inherent instability in the legs because of the joints. Muscles constantly pull on the bones that surround the joints, causing the forces acting on the joints to constantly change. Some have described walking as an act of controlled falling. You are always a few motions away from falling down because of tripping or buckling—yet incredibly you do not! In fact, you are able walk and run—at times even carrying things!

Noted experts in the field of *gait analysis* (the scientific study of walking) believe that some of the major factors in energy conservation during walking involve movements of the pelvis, including pelvic rotations and tilts toward one side.

Walking is divided into two phases—stance and swing. The *stance phase* is the part of the walking cycle that begins when the heel of one foot comes into contact with the ground, and ends when the toes of that same foot push off the ground. In between, the foot gently rolls from initial heel strike to a "foot flat" position before "toe-off." At toe-off, the toes and ball of the foot push up, giving your body the momentum it needs to advance forward.

During *swing phase,* the advancing leg moves forward in space until it is ready to strike the ground with the heel, initiating the heel strike of the stance phase again (Figure 8-1).

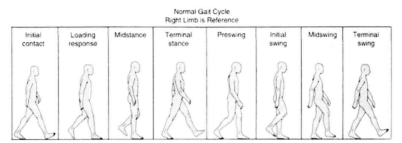

Figure 8-1 Phases of the gait cycle. (From R. Seymour, Prosthetics and Orthotics. Baltimore: Lippincott Williams & Wilkins, 2002. Reprinted by permission of the publisher.)

The speed at which you walk is important. The faster you walk, the more energy is consumed per distance traveled. The slower you walk, the less energy is consumed per distance traveled. Normally we walk at a speed of about 3 miles per hour. At this speed, there is a good balance between the speed of walking and the energy cost required to maintain the speed for long distances.

Pain in the legs or feet alters the way that you walk. This alteration makes the muscles work harder to keep you moving at 3 miles per hour. Your body gets tired faster because the energy cost is higher, and you compensate by walking slower. You will be able to cover the same distance as someone who does not have pain in a limb, but it will take longer.

THE BIOLOGICAL AND BIOMECHANICAL CHALLENGES OF WALKING WITH A PROSTHESIS

Walking is an automatic function. You do not have to think about walking because you have been doing it instinctively since you were about 1 year old. The brain coordinates the act of walking at the subconscious level. The only time you think about walking is when you have pain or limitations, such as an amputation or paralysis. It takes many repetitions to learn how to walk—some say several thousand. Once you are fitted with a prosthesis, you will have to practice many, many times before you get it right!

Losing a limb alters the biomechanics of walking. The absence of a part of your leg decreases your ability to fully control the functions and movements of that limb. This is because the missing muscles and bones previously functioned as a unit. You also lose the sensory feedback that your brain previously received from the missing part. This information was important because it told your brain where your body was in space with respect to the ground. For example, walking on sand is different from walking on concrete. Amputees receive less sensory feedback from the residual limb, depending on which joints are missing (knee and/or ankle). The end result is an unsteady feeling when standing or walking with a prosthesis.

The loss of part of a limb makes the remaining part of the limb the sole surface that is responsible for bearing the weight of the body. Your residual limb was constructed by a surgeon, and it may or may not be up to the challenge that has been imposed on it.

THE RESIDUAL LIMB

As discussed in Chapter 4, the decision as to the level of amputation is based on the condition of the bones, flesh, and blood supply at the time of surgery. The ideal length for a below-the-knee amputation is about one-third of the length of the sound limb. Typically, this is about 6 inches.

There should be enough soft tissue padding at the bottom of the residual limb to protect the hard bones that remain. If the residual limb is too long, there may not be enough soft tissue for padding. It may also be difficult to achieve optimal alignment of the prosthesis. A long residual limb may need less energy to move the limb forward. A short residual limb may have adequate soft tissue padding, but because of its size there will be a great deal of stress placed on it by the hard socket.

It is very important for the surgeon to try and save the knee, but this is not always possible. From a biomechanical point of view, it is also very helpful to have a below-the-knee amputation as opposed to an above-the-knee amputation, because an intact knee can help reduce the energy cost associated with walking.

Alignment of the various prosthetic components with respect to one another is very important. As previously mentioned, the endoskeletal shank is basically a lightweight metal rod that attaches to both the socket and the foot. It can be adjusted at both ends by a prosthetist. A poor fit between the socket and the residual limb may result from poor alignment between the socket and the shank. If this problem is not corrected, it could lead to excessive pressures being placed on the residual limb in the socket. These excessive pressures can cause skin tears and become a source of infection.

SPECIFIC CHALLENGES IN WALKING WITH A PROSTHESIS

The first challenge you will encounter is putting on the prosthesis. Ideally, the residual limb should fit into the socket—like a hand fits into a glove. The fit has to be snug, but not too tight or too loose. This requires a great deal of hand strength, as well as some shifting of the limb until it is inside the socket. You will probably have to put on one or more socks, or a liner, before putting on the prosthesis. You will need more socks if the socket is too big, and fewer socks if the socket is small.

Maintaining your balance will be the next challenge. The physical therapist will teach you how to keep your balance in a variety of settings. At first, this may be between parallel bars in the therapy gym with one or two people standing by your side. Later, it will be with the assistance of a variety of assistive devices, including a walker, crutch, or cane. One of the toughest activities that you will have to master is maintaining your balance when standing, turning, or walking on different surfaces. Some people say that walking sideways down an incline may help to provide greater stability.

It is quite common for amputees to fall. This occurs more often in the initial stages of rehabilitation, while still on the rehab unit. Typically, falling occurs when you become more confident in your abilities and are more active. Some amputees fall while trying to get up in the middle of the night to go to the bathroom because they do not remember that their leg is no longer there. Falling may embarrass you, but can also teach you a valuable lesson—always be aware of your limitations! Falling can be potentially serious, causing fractures, muscle bruises, or head injury. It is extremely valuable to learn how to get up off the floor *before your first fall.* Your therapist can teach you various techniques to accomplish this.

Another common challenge you may encounter as you learn to walk with your prosthesis is muscle and joint pain in the rest of your body. Walking with a prosthesis places greater stress on your unaffected leg. If you are fortunate, that leg will be healthy and able to withstand the added strain. If you have a history of arthritic pain in the knee or hip, however, the added stress may increase your arthritic pain. Let your doctor and therapist know if your pain increases so that they can adjust your therapy program accordingly.

Your doctor can also prescribe pain medications, braces, and cold or warm packs as needed. It is a good idea to take your pain medication about 30 to 45 minutes before you start physical therapy so that you can exercise with greater comfort.

COMMON ABNORMALITIES IN WALKING WITH A PROSTHESIS

Alberto Esquenazi is a leading expert in the analysis of ambulation using a prosthesis. He described some of the common abnormalities noted in people walking with a prosthesis in a 1994 article (10). The remainder of this chapter discusses some of his findings and adds some of the author's own observations.

As previously mentioned, the *gait cycle* is divided into two basic components—swing phase and stance phase. The common problems encountered in walking with a prosthesis can also be divided into these same phases.

Stance Phase Problems with a BK Prosthesis

Problems commonly encountered in the stance phase of walking with a prosthesis include "buckling" of the knee, "snapping back" of the knee, "foot slapping," and "vaulting."

There are several reasons for knee buckling while walking:

- Weak quadriceps: The muscles of the front of your thigh are too weak to help straighten the knee when your heel strikes the ground. This can be corrected by a muscle strengthening program.

- Pain from an ill-fitting socket. Changing the socket might solve this problem.

- A poorly-aligned prosthetic foot, or one with a heel that is too hard. These also can be corrected.

A snapping back sensation can be caused by weak thigh muscles or poor alignment of the socket and the foot. Fear of the knee buckling (which can increase your risk of falling) is offset by keeping the knee as straight as possible when your heel strikes the ground in the early stance phase. One way of keeping it straight is to "snap" the knee back. Over time, this can cause pain and deformity in your knee. A good muscle strengthening program for the thigh muscles is important to overcome this problem.

Additionally, your prosthetist can check the socket to ensure that there is a good fit and alignment.

The foot should also be checked for alignment problems. The knee may snap backwards because of a soft heel or a foot that points downward more than it should.

A prosthetic foot that slaps the floor while walking can be the result of a problem with socket alignment or the foot. For example, there may be a slapping sound if the foot is pointing up too much when the heel strikes the ground. This can also potentially cause the knee to buckle.

Vaulting is the term used when you lift your body up onto the ball of your sound foot in order to swing your prosthetic leg forward. There are a few reasons for vaulting. One is that the prosthesis is too long, and as a result you feel that you are going to trip over it as you walk. You compensate for this by raising your entire body off the ground with your sound foot.

Other reasons include inadequate suspension of the prosthesis or an ill-fitting socket. The end result is the same as if the prosthesis is too long—you compensate by raising your entire body on the ball of your sound foot. These problems can be addressed by correcting the length of the prosthesis, ensuring that the residual limb fits well inside the socket, or adjusting the prosthetic suspension.

Swing Phase Problems with a BK Prosthesis

One leg moves forward during the swing phase of walking. The sound limb and the prosthetic limb alternate. When one is moving forward, the other one is in stance phase. This stabilizes the body so that you do not fall.

The problems encountered during the swing phase of ambulation with a below-the-knee prosthesis are primarily related to an inability to advance the leg. This may be the result of the prosthesis being too long, being inadequately suspended, or having a contracture at the knee, which limits the ability of the knee to bend and straighten effectively.

Pain from a poorly fitting prosthesis or fear of taking steps may affect swing phase. These are all correctible. The length of the prosthesis can be adjusted; the suspension can be improved; the contracture straightened; and the thigh muscles strengthened. If the contracture cannot be straightened, a new socket can be made that will take into account the inability of the knee to fully straighten.

Gait Problems in AK Amputees

According to Alberto Esquenazi, the most common problem encountered by the above-the-knee amputee is bending and straightening the knee during stance phase. You may feel that your knee will buckle and cause you to fall. As a result, you are fearful of walking and take small, cautious steps to compensate. This problem can be corrected by changing the alignment of the knee to make it more stable during stance phase, or your prosthetist may give you a different type of knee—one that emphasizes stability.

There are other reasons for knee-buckling during stance phase that are not related to the use of a prosthesis; for example, weak buttock muscles on the prosthetic limb. This can be remedied by a good muscle strengthening program. Another common problem is having the prosthesis stick out away from the body during stance phase. This is a common result of a muscle imbalance between the muscles that typically pull the prosthetic leg toward the body, and the ones that pull the prosthetic leg away

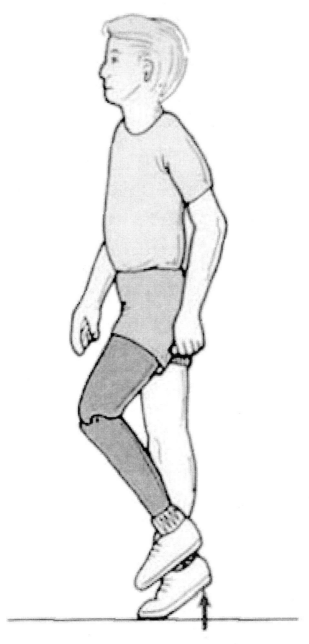

Figure 8-2 Vaulting. (From R. Seymour, Prosthetics and Orthotics. Baltimore: Lippincott Williams & Wilkins, 2002. Reprinted by permission of the publisher.)

from the body. A good muscle strengthening program for the muscle groups that pull the limb toward the body is important.

The prosthetist may recommend an ischial containment socket if you do not already have one. As mentioned previously, this type of socket is narrower in some dimensions, and provides better support to the hip area. Another common problem is too much bending of the trunk during stance phase. This can result from an ill-fitting socket, a short prosthesis, or weak hip muscles.

Vaulting can be seen with an AK prosthesis (in a way similar to the BK prosthesis). It can be caused by a prosthesis that is too long or inadequately suspended (Figure 8-2).

Circumduction is the term that is used to describe a wide arc-like movement of the prosthetic limb during swing phase. Typically, it results from a prosthesis that is too long. The prosthesis may appear to be too long if the suspension is inadequate or the prosthetic knee does not bend (Figure 8-3).

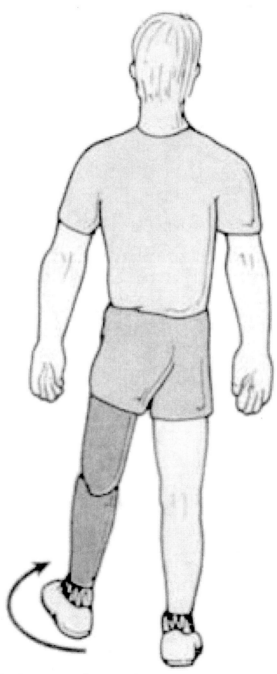

Figure 8-3 Circumducted gait. (From R. Seymour, Prosthetics and Orthotics. Baltimore: Lippincott Williams & Wilkins, 2002. Reprinted by permission of the publisher.)

The Importance of the Hip Muscles

Weakness in the key muscle groups around the hip (the buttock muscles) and contractures or tightness of the hip joint can have a profound impact on your ability to walk with a prosthesis. It can make the way you walk appear awkward and force you to use more energy than you should. You may become overly cautious every time you take a step.

There are four key muscle groups in the area of the hip. Each plays an important role in the ability to walk with a prosthesis:

The *hip flexors* are located in front of the thigh. They are responsible for advancing the leg forward during swing phase. You may find it difficult to advance the limb during swing phase if they are weak.

The *hip extensors* are the buttock muscles. Their job is to help pull the leg backward, stabilizing it during the stance phase. If they are weak, there may be a buckling or un-steady sensation at the time when the pros-thetic heel hits the ground during stance phase.

The *hip abductors* are located on the outside of the hip. Their main function is to pull the leg away from the body. You will walk with an excessive bending of your trunk if they are weak.

The *hip adductors* are located on the inside of the thigh. They pull the prosthetic leg toward the body. You will walk with the prosthetic limb extended away from your body if they are weak.

WEIGHT ISSUES IN WALKING WITH A PROSTHESIS

Weight gain can cause your residual limb to increase in size, making it more difficult to put on a prosthesis. If the prosthesis is not on correctly, chances are that it is not adequately suspended. This can make it more difficult to walk in a smooth, energy-efficient, and attractive manner. It can also cause skin irritations and infections.

People gain weight gain for different reasons, the most common being a sedentary lifestyle. Retaining water from a heart or kidney condition can also be a cause. It is important to discuss any weight gain or loss with your prosthetist and physician. Changes in your prosthesis may be necessary if you are unable to lose weight. These changes may include the fabrication of a new socket.

CORRECTING A SOCKET THAT DOES NOT FIT WELL

An ill-fitting socket can be a source of frustration for patient and prosthetist alike. There are many reasons why a socket may not fit correctly. In addition to weight gain or loss, a thicker liner, use of multiple socks, or improperly putting on these items can also cause problems with fit.

Jennifer Dowell, C.P.O. has written about the additional signs to look for in an ill-fitting prosthesis (11). These include skin irritation, abnormal wear and tear in the gel liner, and abnormal gait.

Excess sweating at rest or with activity, changes in the number of hours that the prosthesis is worn, and changes in the type of activity for which the prosthesis is used can all lead to poor socket fit.

An X-ray of the residual limb with the prosthesis on (while standing) can provide valuable information about socket fit. It can also show any possibly abnormal positions of the thigh bone, which can cause constant friction against the inside aspect of the socket.

Your prosthetist may recommend simple corrections, such as using fewer socks inside the socket or using a thinner gel liner. If none of these work, the prosthetist may try to relieve the point of pressure by using heat or applying pads. Unfortunately, this often relieves the pressure only in one area, while causing increased pressure in another area. Ultimately, you may end up needing a new socket altogether.

Shoes with different heel heights can also cause problems in walking with a prosthesis. The way you walk and the socket fit may be altered if the heel of the shoe on the sound foot is lower or higher than that of the prosthetic shoe.

KEY POINTS

1. Walking with a prosthesis requires more energy than walking with two sound limbs. A person with an above-the-knee amputation requires more energy to walk than a person with a below-the-knee amputation. The higher energy cost is often compensated for by walking slower.

2. Walking is divided in two phases—stance and swing.

3. Key reasons for problems in walking with a prosthesis include:

    • Ill-fitting prosthetic socket

    • Inadequate socket suspension

    • Improper alignment of key prosthetic components (knee or foot)

    • Pain

    • Weak muscles

    • Fear of falling

CHAPTER 9

Returning Home with a Prosthesis

Your transition from the safe confines of the rehab unit to home and the community may present another set of challenges. The hallways of the rehab unit are wide and present few obstacles. There is good lighting, and there is always someone who can help you put on your prosthesis. Everyone is encouraging and takes the time necessary to answer your questions. They work with you at a pace that is comfortable.

Your home may have a smaller living space, narrow hallways, stairs, and inadequate lighting. Small objects may block commonly traveled areas. You may be alone for longer periods of time than you were on the rehab unit.

Many rehab facilities offer a home visit prior to discharge. The home visit is typically performed by an occupational therapist and/or a physical therapist. They will go to your home and assess it for safety risks and make recommendations. They may find that it is not suitable for you to return home because of safety risks. Alternatively (and more commonly), they will offer suggestions for making your home safer. Be sure to take advantage of the home visit if one is offered to you.

Additionally, you may want to ask for a home pass for a few hours during the weekend prior to your discharge to find out how you will manage the everyday issues in your home. Perhaps the front steps to your home are steeper than you remember. Perhaps the wheelchair that you are planning on getting is too wide for the doorways. These are all issues that you can bring back to your rehab team for discussion before you are discharged.

Your significant other may also have concerns and questions about your return home. These should be given equal consideration by the rehab team, because that person will be actively involved in your care once you leave the rehab facility. The most important thing is for you to return to a home that is safe.

HOW TO PREVENT FALLS

As previously mentioned, there is a risk that you may fall at some point after you have had a lower limb amputation. It may happen in the middle of the night when you get up to go to the bathroom because you do not remember that you are missing a leg. Although most of the time nothing serious will happen, there is always the risk that you may break a bone, hit your head, or cut yourself.

First and foremost, it is best to have a safe home that minimizes your risk of falling. Second, you must have a prosthesis that fits well and is not at risk of breaking or malfunctioning. Third, you should know how to get up off the floor if you fall, and how to call for help if you cannot get up off the floor. Your therapists can provide you with more individualized recommendations regarding how to avoid a fall, or how to get up once you have fallen.

Below are some suggestions for modifying your home to prevent falls.

General

1. Remove loose rugs that might slip when you step on them, or make sure that they have an anti-skid mat underneath them. These can be purchased from most carpet stores.

2. Chairs should have arms that make it easy to get up from a sitting position. The legs of the chairs should not stick out because you may trip over them.

3. Tables (including coffee tables) also should not have legs that stick out because you may trip over them.

4. Hallways and other commonly traveled areas in your home should be free of clutter. Examples include stacked magazines, newspapers, bags, and appliances.

5. There should be adequate lighting in all of the living spaces of your home. Light sensors in commonly traveled areas, such as from the bed to the bathroom, can help light up dark areas in the middle of the night so that you do not have to search for a light switch.

6. Have at least one of your phones placed on the floor in a commonly traveled area, so if you fall and cannot reach a phone on a higher surface, you can crawl to the one on the floor.

Specific Rooms

1. **Bathroom:** The bathroom is an area that can pose potential risks for falling. Most bathrooms are small and can be difficult to navigate. In addition, most surfaces are slippery when wet. Some suggestions include:

   • *Grab bars in the tub* should be professionally installed to ensure that they are well anchored to the wall.

   • A *tub bench or seat* can be installed inside the bathtub. These are easily removed. It is a lot easier to wash yourself while sitting down as opposed to standing up.

   • A *handheld showerhead* can be used while sitting on the tub bench. The water temperature can be adjusted while seated.

   • *Adequate lighting* is essential, especially around the medicine cabinet. It is also useful to have a magnifying glass located near your medications. Bottles and pills look alike and can be easily confused.

• *Non-skid mats* should be placed in areas where you anticipate water pooling.

• An *elevated toilet seat* will make it easier to get up off the toilet. A toilet seat that is raised above the usual height with a grab bar nearby can be very useful.

2. **Bedroom**

• Keep a *flashlight* in the nightstand. This can be very useful in the middle of the night or during times of power outage.

• Keeping a *commode or urinal* near your bed can make it easier to empty your bowel or bladder in the middle of the night.

KEY POINTS

1. Having a safe home environment is very important in reducing the risk of falls. Some suggestions for safety include:

• Get rid of loose rugs and use non-skid mats around your home, including the bathroom.

• Commonly traveled areas, such as hallways, should be kept free of clutter and have good lighting.

• Consider bathroom modifications, such as grab bars, tub bench, handheld showerhead, and elevated toilet seat.

CHAPTER 10

Problems Commonly Encountered by Lower Limb Amputees

This chapter discusses the problems that are commonly encountered by lower limb amputees.

SKIN INFECTIONS

Good daily hygiene is very important in preventing skin infections on the residual limb. This is especially important for overweight above-the-knee amputees in the groin area, where the socket comes into contact with the skin. Perspiration, poor hygiene, and constant friction between the socket and the skin can predispose a person to skin infections.

Some general principles of good prosthetic hygiene were outlined by Anne Alexander in a 1975 booklet entitled *Amputee's Guide: Below the Knee* (12), as follows:

- Bathe your leg daily with warm water and soap. Ideally, you should bathe at night.

Bathing in the morning may cause the limb to swell from the warm water, making it more difficult to put on your prosthesis.

- Do not shave the residual limb because this might cause injury to sensitive skin.

- Wash your socks every day with warm water and non-detergent soap. Follow the guidelines of the sock manufacturer.

- Clean the prosthesis socket every day using a damp cloth and mild soap or alcohol.

- Wipe out the insert with a dry cloth every day.

Typically, skin infections occur in the hair roots. The skin will be red and tender to the touch when you have an infection. There may be drainage of liquid material. You may have fever or chills, and not feel well. Notify your physician or nurse at once if any of these conditions occur. If there is a skin break or an infection, you should not wear your prosthesis until it is resolved.

CONTACT DERMATITIS

You may have an allergic skin reaction on your residual limb from the materials used in constructing the components of the socket. Small blisters may appear. If this occurs, do not wear the prosthesis until your doctor has had a chance to look at your skin. Topical medications prescribed by your doctor may be helpful.

CHOKE SYNDROME

As previously mentioned, the socket *must* have total contact with the residual limb. If the top part has total contact and the bottom part does not, then the residual limb will be "choked" at the top. As a result, the venous blood supply in the limb may be compromised. The residual limb may turn purple, have bulging blood vessels, and be swollen. Your prosthetist can modify the socket to correct this condition.

PAIN

Lower limb amputees often experience pain. The most common types include pain in the residual limb, phantom pain, lower back pain, and worsened arthritic pain in the opposite limb.

Residual Limb Pain

There are many reasons for pain in the residual limb, including infection, skin irritation from an ill-fitting socket, pulling on scar tissue at the scar line, or poor circulation in the limb. Sometimes a local nerve may become trapped in the scar tissue, which can cause tingling, shooting pain, and electrical sensations in the residual limb when the tender area is tapped by a finger. This is called a *neuroma.* Various treatments exist for this condition, including injections, medications, socket modification, or acupuncture.

Phantom Pain and Sensation

Phantom pain is one of the mysteries of modern medicine. It is very difficult to comprehend how there can be pain in a part of the body that is no longer there!

The reason that we feel pain after an injury is because the nerve endings in the affected area are stimulated by the injury itself. This sets into motion a series of events that eventually send that message of pain to your brain. The brain then instructs your body to do something about the pain; for example, move the limb away, take a medication, or see a doctor. The more difficult question is: How does part of the body that is no longer there send pain messages to the brain?

One theory revolves around the observation that patients with longstanding pain in the affected limb prior to amputation are at higher risk for phantom pain after amputation. The proposed theory is that the constant pre-surgery pain bombards the brain with so much pain input that after the surgery, the brain can not shut off the stimulation. The result is ongoing pain.

Not all amputees have phantom pain. Many have phantom sensations that their limb is still there, but these sensations are not painful. For example, you may still feel your toes. This is referred to as phantom pain only if the sensation is painful.

Phantom pain has been described as burning, cramping, sharp, electrical, and lancinating. It is often found in amputees who walk less and those who are in poorer health.

No particular treatment has been found to be effective for phantom pain. Some treatments that are commonly used include local electrical stimulation (TENS—transcutaneous electrical nerve stimulation), medications, acupuncture, biofeedback, and skin desensitization techniques, such as tapping the skin.

Musculoskeletal Pain

Low back pain, arthritic flare-up pain in the unaffected limb, and even arm pain have been known to be worsened by the use of a lower limb prosthesis. This is believed to be the result of excessive wear and tear placed on the body as it tries to accommodate to movement with a prosthesis. These are commonly referred to as *overuse injuries.*

It is very important to talk to your doctor and prosthetist about your pain. Sometimes a socket modification, physical therapy, modalities such as heat and cold, a cortisone injection to an arthritic knee, or an anti-inflammatory medication can help reduce your level of discomfort.

KEY POINTS

1. Common problems encountered by a person living with a lower limb amputation include skin infections, pain, and a poorly fitting prosthesis. The risk of skin infections can be minimized by good hygiene. Washing the residual limb, gel liner, and socks daily is very important.

2. Pain is very common in lower limb amputees. The most common types of pain include irritation of the residual limb, phantom pain, and musculoskeletal overuse. It is important to speak to your doctor and prosthetist about any pain you may experience.

CHAPTER 11

Follow-Up Visits to the Rehabilitation Clinic

During your follow-up visits to the rehab clinic, you should tell your doctor if you are experiencing any of the following:

- Areas of redness, cuts, or skin irritations on the residual limb

- Areas of pressure over bones on the residual limb

- Falls or near falls

- Sensations that the residual limb is moving up and down within the socket (pistoning), as opposed to moving *with* the socket. This is similar to walking with a pair of shoes that are too big.

- An ill-fitting prosthesis

- Pain in the residual limb when putting on the prosthesis or taking it off

- Phantom pain

- Low back pain

- Pain in the opposite, remaining lower limb

- A change in the distance you normally ambulate, or the type of terrain

- Problems with respect to dressing, bathing, transferring from bed to chair, or getting in and out of a bathtub

- Any problems with the skin on the opposite foot, such as redness, cuts, and bruises. These are typically on the ball of the foot, and may be difficult to see.

- Any recent weight loss or weight gain

During your follow-up visits, the doctor or other members of the rehab team will typically do the following:

- Examine the residual limb for any evidence of skin problems, such as blisters, infections, or abnormal areas of pressures on bones. The doctor may also examine the skin on your opposite, remaining limb.

- Check the range of motion of the residual limb for the presence of a contracture.

- Examine the strength of your arms and legs, and your ability to get up from a seated position.

- Ask you to ambulate with the prosthesis for a short distance to see if there are any alignment or fit problems with the prosthesis. After this short period of ambulation, your skin will be checked again for any areas of abnormal pressure on the bones.

KEY POINTS

1. Regular follow-up visits to a prosthetic clinic at a rehab center are important. During these visits, the team of rehab professionals will assess your prosthesis for good fit and function. You will also have an opportunity to ask questions and learn about new developments in the field of prosthetics.

CHAPTER 12

The Older, Frail Amputee

This chapter focuses on the key concepts that are of interest to older, frail amputees during rehabilitation, as well as the different prosthetic components available.

Many lower limb amputees are over 65, and have additional medical problems, such as diabetes, heart disease, or circulatory problems. They may have had frequent hospitalizations or admissions to a nursing home or convalescent center in order to treat foot infections or skin breaks in the legs that did not heal. They may have had surgeries in an attempt to improve the circulation in their legs without much success. Ultimately, amputations may have been performed of the toes, foot, or leg.

If you are an older, frail amputee, this has probably been one of the most challenging times of your life. The good news is that there are many other people like you who have been able to successfully adjust to life without a limb. The rehabilitation experts in modern hospitals are very well trained and have many treatment options at their disposal. In addition, a wide range of prosthetic components is available. There are support groups in communities around the country that can help you cope with the challenges ahead.

You may have been significantly weaker when you were transferred to the rehab unit. You may have been sedentary for a long period of time, perhaps sitting in a chair or lying in bed for most of the day. As a result, your muscles and bones have weakened. The muscles and bones need to be used daily in order to stay strong and function well. They become weak without movement, making it difficult to get out of bed.

The most important muscle groups that you need to function in everyday life are the muscles around your shoulders, hands, hips, thighs, and feet—these are pretty much all of the muscles in your body.

The shoulder muscles are responsible for holding up the hands so they can function. Consider the simple act of reaching overhead to a kitchen cabinet to get a cup. You will not be able to reach up to the cabinet if you do not have full motion and strength in your shoulders. As we get older, the shoulders are a common source of pain from arthritis or inflammation of the tendons. These conditions can limit the motion and strength in the shoulders, thereby limiting function.

Our hands are very important. They perform two key functions: (1) touch, feel, and sense objects, and (2) manipulate those objects. Some objects require only a little force to manipulate (a pencil), whereas others require more force (holding the handle of a piece of luggage). The hands are particularly important when putting on a prosthesis or taking it off. Arthritis of the hands can also cause pain and limit function as we get older.

Carpal tunnel syndrome is a condition in which the nerve that travels through the middle of the wrist becomes irritated. This may be the result of diabetes, trauma, or repetitive movements. Subsequently, there can be numbness, tingling in the fingers, and/or weakness in the muscles of the hands.

The muscles that make up your buttocks (also known as *gluteus maximus*) are very important for walking and standing. These muscles weaken very quickly from prolonged sitting or lying down. As a result, it becomes increasingly difficult to stand up from a chair (especially a low one), get on or off a toilet, or in and out of a bed. You may have a difficult time learning how to ambulate with a prosthesis if these muscles are weak.

The quadriceps are an important group of muscles located in the *front* of the thighs. They are responsible for preventing the knees from buckling when walking. The muscles in the *back* of the thighs are known as the *hamstrings.* They bend your knee when you walk.

DIABETES AND REHABILITATION

Diabetes is a very serious illness that can affect many parts of your body—most commonly the brain, heart, kidneys, eyes, blood vessels, and nerves. When diabetes affects the blood vessels and nerves, the result may be a lower limb amputation. The challenge for diabetics will be to learn to use a prosthesis while also coping with the effects of diabetes on the rest of the body. Diabetes can put you at increased risk for stroke or heart attack, limit your eyesight, and diminish your sensation and strength in your hands and remaining limb.

OTHER CHALLENGES FOR THE OLDER, FRAIL AMPUTEE

Other challenges that you may face include the limitations imposed on you by arthritis. Osteoarthritis is a disease of the bones and joints that experts believe may be the result of wear and tear over the course of a lifetime. This is important because, after an amputation, you rely more on your remaining limb for support. It is very common to develop pain in the hip or knee joints of the remaining leg if they are arthritic.

Arthritis can also occur in the back, causing pain. Nerves exit through holes in the vertebrae of your spine. Arthritis can make these holes smaller, leaving less room for the nerves, which, in turn, irritates the nerves and causes further pain. This condition is called *spinal stenosis.*

Typically, people who have this condition complain of low back pain that travels down into the buttocks or calves. The pain is dull, achy, and crampy in nature, and is made worse by standing for a long period of time or walking for a long distance. It is made better by sitting on a chair.

People with spinal stenosis usually avoid certain movements because they may bring on pain. This may be difficult to do when you are learning how to walk with a prosthesis. As a result, there may be a worsening of low back pain.

Problems with your lungs, such as asthma or smoking-related COPD (chronic obstructive pulmonary disease), may be worsened because of the exertion involved in learning to ambulate.

PRECAUTIONS DURING REHAB

The older, frail amputee should undergo the initial phases of rehabilitation in a rehab unit, because the professionals on the unit will be aware of the additional challenges faced by these amputees. They will be able to respond to any possible difficulties the amputee may experience.

Rehabilitation prescriptions have certain built-in precautions that therapists must abide by. This includes the special precautions to be taken with cardiac and pulmonary patients, and for amputees who are more likely to fall. They are also trained to watch for side effects of medications. Cardiac precautions are meant to set upper limits on the amount of stress placed on your heart as you perform your exercises. Typically, the therapist measures your blood pressure and pulse, and notifies your physician if these values are above or below a certain number. Your therapist may also periodically ask you during an exercise how hard you are exerting yourself. Ideally, you should be able to talk comfortably while exercising. If you find it difficult to talk, it probably means that you are overexerting yourself and should slow down.

Pulmonary precautions are meant to give your therapist an indication of how fast you are breathing while exercising. Normally, you should breathe about 20 times per minute. Anything more frequent than that may indicate either a medical problem or overexertion. Sometimes a therapist may put a small clamp known as a *pulse oximeter* on your finger. This device gives a reading that measures the oxygen level of your blood. The therapist relies on this number to indicate how well your blood is being oxygenated while you exercise.

Falls are a common concern for people with amputations. As mentioned earlier, older, frail amputees are at a higher risk for falling when they are first learning to walk with a prosthesis. This is a realistic concern, and your therapist will take every precaution to advance your training with a prosthesis at a pace that is comfortable and safe.

LEARNING TO WALK WITH A PROSTHESIS

In the beginning, you will practice standing between two parallel bars with one or two therapists by your side. Later, you will walk between the parallel bars while focusing on coordinating the motions of your prosthetic limb and sound limb. Once you are deemed safe to ambulate outside of the parallel bars, you will gradually progress to using a walker, forearm crutches, and eventually a single cane or perhaps no assistive device at all. Determine the assistive device that you feel the safest with and then stick with it—whether it is a walker, crutch, or cane. Your therapist can also show you some techniques of getting up from the floor if you fall.

PROSTHETIC COMPONENTS FOR LIMITED AMBULATORS

Safety, stability, and ease of use are the main principles that guide decision-making regarding which prosthetic components should be used for an older, frail amputee. The prosthesis must be safe and stable when you are transferring from one surface to another (such as from a wheelchair to a bed), walking on different surfaces (indoor and outdoor), walking at different speeds, and up and down the stairs.

Ideally, the prosthesis should also be light in weight and easy to put on and take off. Adequate suspension can be a challenge for older amputees because of fluctuating residual limb size (for example, from dialysis or congestive heart failure), or painful arthritic joints. Pin-and-lock gel liner systems are often prescribed, but additional socks may also be added or removed to accommodate the change in residual limb size. Secondary systems, such as a thigh cuff, may also be needed to ensure adequate suspension.

The type of prosthetic foot chosen depends on how and where you plan on using the prosthetic limb. A SACH foot may be adequate if you are limited in your ability to walk. A lightweight, energy-storing foot may be more appropriate if you are a more active walker who does not engage in strenuous physical activities. The prosthetic knee is crucial in providing support and stability at the most critical point of the walking cycle for above the knee amputees. This is the time when the foot of the prosthetic limb comes into contact with the ground. At this point, the knee could buckle, causing a fall. Stance-control knees, polycentric knees, and the manual-locking knee have all been used to address this problem. Each type of knee has advantages and disadvantages.

It is *always* important to ensure that the prosthesis can be put on and taken off with relative ease. Impaired vision and hands that have been weakened by arthritis or nerve damage can make this task difficult. Sometimes, prosthetists will attach hooks made out of canvas material to the socket components to make the prosthesis easier to put on or take off. Family members and friends should also be taught how to properly attach the prosthesis to the residual limb. You may have an ill-fitting socket if putting on the prosthesis becomes more and more difficult. As mentioned earlier, this may be the result of change in the size of the residual limb or a recent weight gain or loss.

KEY POINTS

1. The older amputee may be weak from multiple hospitalizations prior to the amputation surgery. The amputee may face additional challenges related to poor vision,

diabetes, arthritic pain, and heart and/or lung problems.

2. Rehabilitation programs for older, frail amputees are designed with these limitations in mind, and precautions are used while performing exercises.

3. Safety, stability, and ease of application are the most important principles in prescribing prosthetic components for the older, frail amputee.

CHAPTER 13

The Bilateral Amputee

The number of people living with two lower limb amputations (also known as *bilateral amputations*) has been steadily rising. Living with two amputations poses significant challenges, but there are many reported cases of people who have overcome the odds and found a way to live a full and productive life. This chapter briefly describes some of these challenges and offers suggestions on how to address them.

To begin with, not all bilateral amputees are the same. Some people may have one below-the-knee amputation and a second partial foot amputation. Others may have two below-the-knee amputations, and still others may have two above-the-knee amputations.

Although there are practical differences among them, they all share four unique challenges:

- Increased energy expenditure for ambulation

- Decreased balance

- The need for strong arms and trunk muscles

- The need for at least one assistive device, such as a walker, crutch, or cane

INCREASED ENERGY REQUIREMENTS

The higher the level of amputation of both legs, the more energy will be required for ambulation—sometimes as much as two to three times more—as compared to a person who does not have an amputation. This makes walking very difficult, especially if you have other medical conditions, such as heart or lung disease.

Because of the high energy cost of walking, many bilateral amputees rely a great deal on walking aids, such as walkers, crutches, or canes. You should use the walking device that makes you feel the safest.

Wheelchairs are commonly used by bilateral amputees for both household and community mobility. This is perfectly reasonable, because you should not have to expend all your energy getting from one place to another, and then be exhausted once you get there.

There are many types of wheelchairs, but not all of them are good for the bilateral amputee.

The *amputee wheelchair* is one that has certain built-in features that make it easier and safer for use by an amputee. One of these features is a wheel axle that is set more toward the back of the chair. This makes it less likely that it will tip backwards. Other features include removable arm rests and swing-away leg rests. These make it easier to perform transfers from one surface to another.

Power wheelchairs can make a significant difference in the lives of bilateral amputees who are very active. This type of wheelchair can make it easier to maintain a high level of mobility in the community, when combined with appropriately adapted vans or minivans.

LOSS OF BALANCE

Loss of balance is always a problem for the bilateral amputee who walks with two prostheses, especially if the legs are amputated at different levels. The prosthetic components used for bilateral amputees are meant to emphasize safety and stability. This may include wider feet, polycentric knees, and auxiliary suspension devices, just to name a few.

Nevertheless, if you are planning to walk with two prostheses, you will need to devote a considerable amount of your rehabilitation to balance training.

THE IMPORTANCE OF GOOD TRUNK AND ARM STRENGTH

Good arm and trunk muscle strength is necessary to qualify for bilateral prosthetic limbs, because bilateral amputees rely a great deal on their arms and trunk. Prior to being considered for prosthetic limbs, your doctor, prosthetist, or physical therapist may recommend a strengthening program. This could be as an inpatient on a rehabilitation unit in a medical center or as an outpatient.

PROSTHESES ARE NOT ALWAYS NECESSARY

Not all bilateral amputees need or want prosthetic limbs. If you decide that it is too difficult to learn to use two prostheses, or it requires too much energy to walk with them, then you should take comfort in knowing that many bilateral amputees resort to other ways of getting around their homes. Using their hands for assistance, they move around on their knees, buttocks, or residual limbs. There is an increased risk of skin irritation when doing this, but it can be minimized by using knee pads or well padded pants.

HIP CONTRACTURES

As a bilateral amputee, you probably spend a great part of your time in the sitting position. This may be on a bed, a wheelchair, or the floor. As a result, the muscles around your hips can become tight and possibly even contract into a fixed position. This may make it more difficult to walk with prostheses. Therefore, it is important to perform good stretching exercises for these muscles. A good way to prevent contractures of the hip muscles is to spend some part of your day lying flat on your stomach. Your physical therapist can also show you stretching exercises that will help prevent contractures.

STUBBIES

Stubbies are short prostheses prescribed for bilateral transfemoral amputees. They can be very functional when used around the house, because they are low to the ground and are much steadier than traditional prostheses. They also require less energy to use (Figure 13-1).

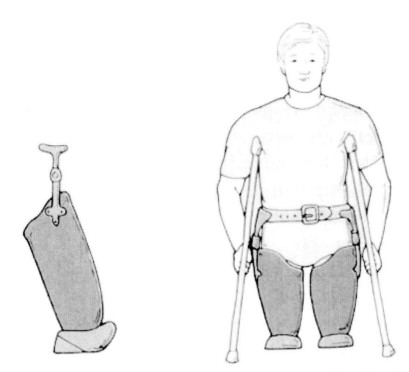

Figure 13-1 Stubbies may be used by individuals with bilateral transfemoral amputations. They are more stable than regular prostheses because the center of gravity is lowered. (From R. Seymour, Prosthetics and Orthotics. Baltimore: Lippincott Williams & Wilkins, 2002. Reprinted by permission of the publisher. The figure was originally adapted from O'Sullivan, S.B. & Schmitz, T.J. [1994]. Physical Rehabilitation: Assessment and Treatment [3rd ed.]. Philadelphia, PA: F.A. Davis.)

KEY POINTS

1. Bilateral amputees expend a considerable amount of energy when walking.

2. Not all bilateral amputees need or want to walk with two prostheses.

3. Walking with two prostheses requires good balance, and arm and trunk strength.

4. Stubbies are short prostheses for bilateral transfemoral amputees that can be a very functional alternative to traditional prostheses.

CHAPTER 14

The Child with a Lower Limb Amputation

A national survey carried out in 1975 found that most cases of amputation in children are the result of trauma or cancer. In addition, some children are born with a limb or part of a limb that is either absent or deformed. These are known as *congenital deformities.* The most common congenital deformity of the lower limb is an absence of the *fibula,* one of the two bones that make up the calf. This condition can lead to a bow-shaped deformity of the calf, which is often associated with a shortened leg.

The other bone of the calf (known as the *tibia*) may also be absent or malformed. This is important because this bone is responsible for bearing the weight of the body when the child is standing or walking.

Another possible congenital deformity is the partial absence of a part of the thigh bone at its attachment to the hip. As a result, the leg is shortened and often malrotated. This may also be associated with an unstable knee joint.

THE IMPACT OF AMPUTATION ON DEVELOPMENT OF THE CHILD

The most important thing to remember about children who are born without a limb—or who have lost a limb because of an accident or illness—is that they are first and foremost children, not small adults.

In some ways, having an amputation as a child is easier than as an adult. Children generally have good health; they have a tremendous amount of energy; they are quick learners; and they are typically less fearful of learning new things than adults.

The adult with an amputation often has many other medical problems, more limited energy, and may have difficulty learning complex concepts, such as walking with a prosthesis. According to Ellen Leonard (13), children require little training in the use of a lower limb prosthesis. Play is the most important activity of the day for children, and they learn quickly if the training is incorporated into a play activity.

Self-image and acceptance by family and friends are very important to a child, and the use of a prosthesis can adversely impact their emotional and psychological development.

FITTING A CHILD WITH A PROSTHESIS

A child begins to stand and walk between the ages of 9 and 12 months. This is the ideal time to fit the child with a first prosthesis. The child is just learning how to balance on two legs, making it easier to accept the prosthesis.

Children grow quickly, primarily in height. The sound limb and the remaining parts of the limb with the deformity or amputation also grow. Therefore, it is recommended that a child be fitted with a new prosthesis once each year between the ages of 1 and 5; every 2 years between the ages of 6 and 12, and every 3 to 4 years between the ages of 13 to 21. A new prosthesis may be needed more frequently during periods of accelerated growth.

THE NEED FOR MODIFICATION BECAUSE OF RAPID GROWTH

The bones of children tend to grow more in length than in width, but both types of growth need to be considered when fabricating the prosthesis. Placing a soft pad at the bottom of the socket when the limb is still small is a good idea. This pad can be removed as the child grows.

Substituting a short endoskeletal shank for a longer one as the child grows is another modification. Thicker socks can also be worn inside the socket. As the child's limb grows in circumference, fewer and thinner socks can be used to accommodate the growth.

Nevertheless, if you have a child who has an amputation, it is important for you to recognize the signs that the prosthesis does not fit well:

- The child complains of pain when using the prosthesis.

- It gets progressively more difficult to put on the prosthesis.

- The skin is red or has tears.

It is a good idea to have three to four checkups each year with the prosthetist, and two with the rehab physician to ensure that the prosthesis is the right size for the child. Typically, the child will probably need a new prosthesis every 1 to 3 years during the peak growing years.

DIFFERENCES IN PROSTHESES FOR CHILDREN AND ADULTS

Children are very active, and will use the prosthesis during many physical activities, such as running and jumping. They may not be very diligent about maintaining the prosthesis in an optimal condition. Believe it or not, this is all right. You should expect the prosthesis to be somewhat worn if the child plays actively. It is more of a concern if the child is not using the prosthesis, and it just sits in a closet in perfect condition.

The components used for the first lower limb prosthesis should emphasize safety, while still allowing the child to engage in age-appropriate activities. More sophisticated components can be used as the child masters ambulation on different surfaces. For example, a hydraulic knee and a sophisticated energy-conserving foot may be appropriate for a highly active teenager, but not for a young child or toddler. A child under 2 years of age is too young to learn how to use a prosthetic knee joint. As a result, the child may fall frequently because she does not know how to keep the knee stable while walking. Therefore, it is recommended that children be fitted with a prosthesis that does not have a knee joint until they are older and can understand the appropriate way to use it. Also, the more gadgets that are included on the prosthesis, the heavier it is to wear.

Typically, an endoskeletal shank is prescribed because it can be adjusted more readily than an exoskeletal shank. An exoskeletal shank should be considered if durability is important. This might be the case if the child lives in a remote area, and it is difficult for him to come in for adjustments.

Once a child is developmentally mature enough to understand the use and care of a prosthesis, the child can benefit from the same components that adults use. For example, the suction suspension system is very good, but it requires that the child have good strength and hand dexterity. A young child may not possess the skill and strength to put the suction socket on, but an older child or teenager probably will.

THE CHILD WITH AN ABOVE-THE-KNEEAMPUTATION

A good choice of suspension for the child with an above-the-knee amputation is either the

Silesian belt or the total elastic suspension system. Once the child has good hand dexterity and strength, he can be switched to a suction or silicone suspension system. This is usually at about 6 to 7 years old.

The manual-locking knee is a good choice for a toddler who is just beginning to walk because it provides very good stability. As you may recall from Chapter 7, this type of knee is kept locked until the individual pulls on a cable or presses a button, allowing the knee to bend.

Older children (aged 8 and above) can benefit from a hydraulic knee because they are more active and need a knee that can accommodate walking at different speeds. The disadvantages of this type of knee are that they are heavier and they require more maintenance.

DIFFICULTIES FOR CHILDREN WITH AMPUTATIONS

Children do not have problems with phantom pain or pain from nerves trapped in scar tissue as often as adults. Contractures around the hip or knee are also not as common as they are in adults. One problem that is more common in children is *overgrowth of bone* in the remaining part of the amputated limb. As mentioned earlier, the bones of children grow in both length and circumference. There is a risk that the growing bones in the remaining part of the amputated limb will put pressure on the softer muscles surrounding them. This can be a source of pain for the child, and may limit the child's use of the prosthesis. There is also the risk that the bone may actually push through the skin. (This is more common in the calf bones.) One way to prevent this is to perform the amputation surgery directly through the knee, rather than through the bones above or below it. This is called a *knee disarticulation.* It makes it easier for the residual limb to bear the weight of the body, as well as to suspend the prosthesis.

If the amputation surgery has to be through the long shaft of a bone, the surgeon may consider putting a "cap" of transplanted bone on the end of the remaining part of the amputated bone to prevent further growth.

Another problem that often occurs is *uneven leg length* between the bones of the sound limb and those of residual limb. Initially, this may not be a big issue, but it can become more important as the child grows. The small difference in limb length noted in early childhood may become quite large by the time the child is a teenager. Various tables and figures are used to predict what the eventual leg length difference will be. Once that is determined, a combination of various surgical procedures and prostheses can be used to address uneven leg length.

Some of these surgeries may consist of further amputation or reconstructions. Sometimes a leg-lengthening procedure may be helpful. This often necessitates the placement of a transplanted piece of muscle and/or skin over the lengthened bone. The timing of surgery is important. Children experience less psychological trauma from the loss of a limb if the surgery is performed before the age of 2.

The goal is always the same: to provide the child with a functional, cosmetic residual limb and an energy-efficient prosthesis.

REHABILITATION AND CHILDREN

There is not much of a difference in the rehabilitation of an older child or teenager with an amputation than an adult with a similar below-the-knee or above-the-knee amputation.

There is a pre-prosthetic phase during which the muscles of the arms, the sound limb, and the remaining part of the amputated limb are strengthened. During this phase, shaping of the residual limb with bandage wrappings and shrinkers is also carried out. Most children with amputations are in fairly good health, and are able to complete the preprosthetic phase fairly quickly.

The first prosthesis that the child receives usually has components emphasizing safety in order to minimize the risk of falling. The child learns to walk with the prosthesis on different surfaces (indoors and outdoors) as well as stairs, and progresses from walking between parallel bars in a rehab gym to using an assistive device, such as a walker or crutches. Eventually, the child may become proficient enough to only use a straight cane or perhaps no assistive device at all.

The initial prosthetic training is usually carried out on the rehabilitation unit of a medical center or children's hospital. This is continued in an outpatient setting after the child has returned home.

It is important for the child to receive the initial rehabilitation care from an experienced team of rehabilitation experts. This team usually consists of a physiatrist (a physician who specializes in rehabilitation medicine), physical therapist, occupational therapist, recreational therapist, rehabilitation nurse, prosthetist, psychologist, and social worker. This type of team is typically located in large medical centers, rehabilitation hospitals, or children's hospitals.

The newborn child with a congenital deformity may have additional deformities, and it is important to have the child thoroughly evaluated by a knowledgeable physician. This specialist may want to evaluate the child's limbs and spine with X-rays or other radiological procedures, as well as examine siblings and other family members.

The child's early prosthesis should be age-appropriate, and it should be incorporated into play activities because this is how children explore the world. The prosthesis should be seen as an aid in the child's development.

KEY POINTS

1. A child is not a miniature adult.

2. The most common causes for amputations in children and teenagers are trauma and cancer. Some children are born with con-

genital deformities, such as missing or malformed limbs.

3. Children have a great amount of energy and are quick learners. Learning to walk with a prosthesis may be easier for them than for adults.

4. Children are self-conscious about their appearance, and acceptance by their friends and family is very important to them.

5. A child's developmental stages should be taken into account when prescribing a prosthesis.

6. Children grow quickly and need new prostheses frequently. There are various techniques that can be used to extend the life of a prosthesis.

CHAPTER 15

Sports and the Lower Limb Amputee

There are many advantages to exercising regularly, including benefits to the heart, muscles, and bones, as well as the mind. Just because you have a lower limb amputation does not mean that you cannot participate in athletic activities! This chapter describes some of the advances in prosthetic design that can enable you to participate in a variety of sports. Specific concerns to be considered when exercising with a lower limb prosthesis are also discussed.

The expressed interest of amputees in being able to jump and run farther and faster is the major reason for the wide selection of prosthetic components that are available. These amputees do not want to be sidelined while everyone else around them participates in sporting events. As a result, the prosthetics industry has come out with numerous prosthetic improvements, including the concept of energy-storing feet, which was discussed in Chapter 7.

If you are an amputee who is interested in exercising, there are several issues that you need to think about and discuss with your prosthetist:

- What kind of sport do you want to participate in? The demands placed on the prosthetic limb are different if you are a runner versus a golfer.

- Do you plan on using the prosthesis primarily for athletic activities, or for a combination of daily walking at the office and weekend hiking? The prosthetist can recommend a socket with interchangeable foot and shank components if you plan on using the prosthesis for a combination of activities.

- How much stability will you need for your athletic activity? This is important if you enjoy hiking or playing basketball. Both of these activities place great stress on the knee. The prosthetist can recommend a thigh cuff suspension that will provide greater stability. If you have a transfemoral amputation, there are certain types of prosthetic knees that can provide you with greater stability when you need it most.

- If you are a runner, do you plan on running fast or slow? Some prosthetic feet come with a built-in shock absorber that can dampen the stress placed on the residual limb. This is accomplished by attaching the foot directly to the socket.

The socket is very important in sporting activities. It transmits a substantial force to the residual limb as you run, hike or jump. The socket has to provide a very tight fit and be fabricated from lightweight materials. The force of the impact can cause damage to the skin, muscles, and bones of the residual limb if the fit is not good. A silicone suction suspension system can often protect the skin from these forces.

The choice of prosthetic knee can be very important for sports such as running. A hydraulic knee can be quite useful for this type of activity. Knees with built-in microprocessors are available; for example, the *C-leg* by Otto Bock Orthopedic Industry Inc. (see Figure 7-4 in CHAPTER 7). The main advantage of this type of knee is that it allows running at different speeds and up and down inclines.

Some sports, including golf, require a great deal of trunk and limb rotation. In such cases, a *rotator* can be attached to the prosthesis. This device allows the prosthesis to turn while the foot remains flat on the ground, reducing the amount of friction in the area where the socket comes into contact with the residual limb.

Water sports pose unique challenges because prosthetic components are usually not waterproof. Serious damage can result to the prosthesis if you submerge it under water, especially saltwater. The prosthesis can be made waterproof by covering it with a special material. There are also special swimming prostheses that can be purchased.

THE UNIQUE CHALLENGES OF RUNNING, CYCLING, SWIMMING, AND GOLF

Running, cycling, swimming, and golf are very common activities engaged in by lower limb amputees. They each have their own unique challenges.

Running

Running is difficult for an amputee to master. It requires strong thigh and buttock muscles, as well as good balance. Substantial impact force is generated during running. This force gets transmitted to both the prosthetic limb and the residual limb. This can be a source of pain in the residual limb, hip, and even the lower back. There may also be a considerable amount of friction between the socket and the residual limb. This can be minimized by a socket that fits well, a gel liner, and direct attachment of the prosthetic foot to the socket itself.

You may want to consider walking at a brisk pace if you find that running is too difficult. This can be performed at a school track, a neighborhood park, or even on a treadmill. Just keep in mind that the harder the surface, the greater the stress of the impact. Also, keep in mind that uneven terrains, such as a grass field or sand, can pose unique balance challenges.

Cycling

Cycling is a very good form of exercise that can be performed in your home on a stationary bicycle, or on a regular bicycle out in the community. There are two unique challenges posed by riding a bicycle in the community: (1) a considerable amount of balance is required to get on and off a bicycle. A few training sessions with a physical therapist in the proper technique of mounting a bicycle can be very beneficial. (2) There is a risk of potential trauma to the residual limb. This risk is present regardless of whether a prosthesis is worn or not during cycling. Transfemoral amputees may have pain when sitting on a hard bicycle seat while wearing a prosthesis. You may want to consider purchasing a wider, softer seat if you are an avid cyclist. Your prosthetist might also be able to fabricate a socket with a softer, more flexible rim. He may suggest a prosthesis that attaches directly to the bicycle pedal.

Golf

The major challenge faced in golf is maintaining your balance while swinging the club, because your feet need to remain on the ground while the rest of your body turns. This can be especially difficult if you are a transfemoral amputee. As mentioned earlier, a rotator can be of help, but you should consider working with your physical therapist on balance and the proper swing. Your therapist might also recommend a golf clinic for amputees in your area, where you can perfect your game with assistance. Another challenge is walking with a prosthesis on the uneven terrain of a golf course. Consider using a golf cart to get around the course if you find it too difficult to navigate.

Swimming

In many ways, swimming is an ideal sport if you are an amputee. It eliminates the harsh impact associated with other sports, such as running. The buoyancy of the water helps reduce the stress on the hip, knee, and lower back. It can also be performed with or without a prosthesis.

The major challenge associated with swimming is getting in and out of the water. A considerable amount of balance and strength is required to accomplish this task. Walking in water may also be a problem when swimming in the ocean because of uncertain foot placement on the sandy ocean floor.

As mentioned earlier, swimming prostheses and waterproof covers for existing prostheses can make it easier to enjoy swimming. It is also helpful to use a non-skid shoe to prevent falls when walking in or around the water. A few sessions with a physical therapist can be helpful in learning how to get in and out of the water at the pool.

EXERCISING PRECAUTIONS

Some good rules to observe while exercising include:

Always Check the Skin on the Residual Limb

This is especially important *after* activity. Exercising with an ill-fitting prosthesis can cause injury to the skin. The sound limb may also be at risk if you wear an inappropriate shoe and have poor sensation and circulation in that foot.

Check with the Doctor before Beginning an Exercise Program

As mentioned earlier, some of the most common causes of amputation include peripheral vascular disease and complications associated with diabetes. These conditions can also affect other parts of your body, including your heart. Your doctor can prescribe a stress test to determine how hard you should exercise, and help you create a safe exercise program based on the results of the test.

Be Careful in Choosing a Sport

Depending on your type of amputation and your medical condition, some sports may not be appropriate, and can predispose you to injury. Walking is a good type of exercise because it can be done anywhere and does not need any special equipment or additional training beyond the initial prosthetic training. Swimming is also a good sport to consider.

Listen to Your Body

You should be able to carry on a conversation with someone while you exercise. If you find this to be difficult, then you may be exercising too hard and need to slow down. You should not have pain after you exercise. Pain is typically an indication that you pushed yourself too hard and need to decrease the intensity of your exercise routine. Pain in the residual limb after exercising may be an indicator of an ill-fitting socket, and should be checked by your doctor.

Wear Appropriate Clothing

You should wear loose, comfortable clothing while exercising. Wear an appropriate shoe on the sound limb. This will prevent injury to the foot.

Exercise at a Time of Day that is not Subject to Extreme Weather

Avoid exercising in very hot or very cold weather, because this can place additional stress on your body. Choose a time of day when you realistically think you will be able to exercise on a regular basis.

Exercise with a Friend

One of the most difficult things to do is to exercise alone. You may be more motivated if you exercise with a friend, who might be able to help you if a problem arises.

Exercise Most Days of the Week for about 20 to 30 Minutes Each Day

Consider a supervised exercise program that is monitored by a therapist or physician if your balance is impaired, or if you have a medical problem, such as diabetes or heart disease.

KEY POINTS

1. Exercising with a prosthetic limb poses specific challenges. It is important to communicate clearly with your prosthetist about how you plan on using the prosthesis.

2. Adaptations to the prosthetic socket, knee, and foot can be made that will enable you to participate in specific athletic activities.

3. It is important to undergo a medical evaluation prior to starting an athletic activity program.

4. Always check the skin on your residual limb after exercising.

CHAPTER 16

Coping with the Loss of a Limb

The loss of a limb is one of the most significant challenges that you will ever encounter. It is different from any of the other illnesses and struggles that you may have had, because it is a highly visible, physical loss. You are reminded of it each time that you get dressed. It has an effect on your mobility, and can also have an impact on your hobbies, work, and independence.

This chapter addresses some of these challenges, and offers ways to cope and flourish in spite of them. These suggestions and observations are a combination of the author's own experiences in caring for people with amputations as well as information from the writings of David Fordyce and Lance E. Trexler (14).

THE EMOTIONAL CHALLENGES

If you are similar to most amputees, you were not at your best when the doctors told you that you were going to lose a limb. Chances are that you were acutely ill, hospitalized, and in pain. Also, you were probably weak from having been confined to your bed for a long period of time.

Post-surgical pain, limited mobility, poor appetite, poor sleep, and weakness from pro-longed bedrest had probably made you feel anxious, sad, and fearful. Concerns about your health, your family, and your future may have been overwhelming. At times, you probably felt that you were on an emotional rollercoaster. These are all legitimate feelings to have after the ordeal of amputation surgery.

Experts tell us that there is tremendous variability in the way that people cope with illness. What gets one person through a major health crisis may not help another and vice versa. Each person handles a crisis differently because every person's life experiences are different. If you have spent the past several months in and out of hospitals undergoing painful procedures and surgeries in an attempt to save your leg, you may view the amputation with relief, knowing that your suffering will cease and you can get on with your life. On the other hand, if you were in good health until an accident made it necessary for you to have an amputation, you may be in shock at your loss and saddened by your condition.

Most importantly, *there is no right or wrong way to feel after an amputation.* This is a very personal experience.

Emotional Challenges on the Rehab Unit

As discussed in previous chapters, you will undergo rehabilitation after your amputation, including learning how to use a prosthesis. The rehab unit will not be a very private place. There will always be someone who tries to tell you what to do, how to feel, or inadvertently minimizes your emotions in order to encourage you to work on practical challenges.

Rehabilitation does not allow much time for self-pity. You will only have a short period of time on the unit during which to learn how to care for yourself. This typically means bathing, dressing, feeding, and walking. You will be very busy with a multitude of activities while you are on the unit, including physical therapy, occupational therapy, and recreational therapy. There will be numerous meetings with doctors, social workers, and psychologists.

When you finally find a few minutes to relax in your room, a nurse, a nurse's aide, or a janitor may come in to give you medications or clean your room. Even if you feel depressed, fearful, or anxious, you will not have much time or privacy to dwell on these feelings while you are on the rehab unit.

Unfortunately, the rehab staff may not have had adequate training to address your emotional needs. Most physical or occupational therapists do not have a great deal of psychological training as part of their curriculum. The same can be said for doctors, whose training in this area is often limited.

Chances are that your therapists and doctors are younger than you. Their relatively younger age may make them less likely to understand the impact of your loss, or it may make them feel uncomfortable discussing your emotions. They are often significantly pressured to see many patients in the course of a day. As a result, they may focus on only the practical aspects of your rehabilitation and minimize the emotional component.

Emotional Challenges at Home

Going home will also present emotional challenges. It is one thing to spend several weeks on a rehabilitation unit—where there are other amputees and people who will take care of you—but it is quite another to be back in your home. Everyone moves at a faster pace in the "real world," and may not be as understanding or sympathetic to your emotional concerns.

Your family may also be anxious and concerned about your return home. They may feel that they do not have the practical skills to help you. They may not understand your limitations, or what you are capable of doing. They may feel awkward about approaching you with specific questions or concerns, because they do not want to upset you or themselves. *These are normal feelings.* Remember, there is no right or wrong way to feel after an amputation. This goes for family members and friends as well.

COPING STRATEGIES

Having outlined some of the emotional challenges, as well as some of the inherent difficulties in the rehabilitation process, there are many things that you can do to cope and flourish in spite of the difficulties. The next section discusses some coping strategies:

Express Your Concerns

Everything about the experience of amputation is probably is foreign to you. It is only natural that you will have a great number of questions and concerns. Share them with the rehab staff. They have treated many patients with amputations, and will try to answer your questions. They are not mind-readers, however. If your favorite hobby is hiking in the mountains, they probably will not anticipate questions on this subject unless you ask them. Voice your concerns in a pleasant, nonconfrontational manner. For example, let your therapists know if you become fatigued from the timing of your physical and occupational therapy sessions so they can change your schedule.

You should also take advantage of regular team meetings while you are an inpatient on the rehab unit. The majority of the treating staff will be present at these meetings, and any concerns you have can be addressed.

Be an Active Participant in Your Rehabilitation

What you get out of rehabilitation is directly related to what you invest in it. You will be at a disadvantage if you do not fully participate in the rehab program while you are on the rehab unit. Your insurance company may have placed a limit on the total number of days you can stay on the unit, so make the best of your time. If you do not take full advantage of your time on the unit, you will miss out on a valuable opportunity to receive individualized therapy from a team of professionals.

Always ask questions, especially regarding information about outside resources. If your hobby is going to the theatre, and you are concerned about public transportation and wheelchair accessibility, talk to the recreational therapist in your rehab facility.

Carry a Notebook at All Times

Always carry a notebook and a pencil. Think of rehab as school, and the doctors, nurses, and therapists as your teachers. Write down your questions in the notebook, and identify the therapists who are in the best position to answer them. Keep a written record of the advice you receive during rehabilitation so that you can refer to it later at home.

Gather as Much Information as Possible

There is a wealth of information available on the Internet, including Web sites devoted to amputees and amputee resources. There are also support groups made up of amputees just like you. These groups can be a great source of valuable information. Your recreational therapist, prosthetist, or physical therapist can also be sources of information.

Denial Is Not Necessarily Bad

In the immediate period after your amputation surgery, you may find that it is too emotionally painful to come to grips with the fact that you have lost a limb. *This is entirely understandable.* Everyone grieves differently, and there is no right way or wrong way to feel after such a life-altering event. At first, you may deny the full extent of your problems—both to yourself and to others. This is not necessarily a bad thing.

The Glass Is Half Full ... You Are Lucky to Be Alive

Keep in mind that the limb had to be amputated in order to save your life. This approach might be helpful when you are feeling down. If you believe that you will walk again ... well, then, maybe it will make you work harder! The author has had numerous patients who did not seem to be good candidates for using a prosthesis, but he was happily proven wrong by determined, motivated individuals who wanted to walk again. You might not be able to run a marathon 1 month after a below-the-knee amputation, but it does not hurt to work toward that goal if it will get you out of your rehab bed and into the gym. Always listen to your rehab team. They know what you realistically can and cannot do.

Develop a Quality Relationship with at Least One Therapist

Develop a good working relationship with at least one member of the rehabilitation team. This relationship will make it easier for you to progress through rehab, and allay your fears and concerns as they arise. It does not matter if the therapist is young and inexperienced or a seasoned professional, as long as you develop a mutual bond. Remember, there is a great deal you can learn from each other!

Have Realistic Expectations

No matter how advanced the field of prosthetics becomes, your prosthesis will never be as good as your leg used to be. At best, it is a pretty good approximation. The fit may not always be the way you want it to be. It may be too loose or too tight. You may find that it becomes more difficult to put the prosthesis on or take it off if you gain weight. Raise realistic concerns with your prosthetist, but remember he is not a magician. He is limited by the tools and technology that are available.

So do not expect to run ten blocks soon after getting your prosthesis, if prior to your amputation you could only walk a block before becoming tired.

Focus on New Ways of Performing Tasks

Rehabilitation medicine is a very practical branch of medicine. As a result, the therapists, doctors, and engineers who work in this field are often very creative in solving problems.

Their goal is always to maximize function. For example, an item known as a *reacher* may be suggested if you have difficulty reaching for an object on a high shelf. This is basically a rod with a claw-like device at one end that can hold an object in its grip.

Another example is the *motorized wheelchair* or *power scooter.* If walking with a prosthesis is too slow, or if you fatigue quickly while walking, then one of these devices might be right for you. You will be able to get around the community much more quickly and spend less energy on walking if you use a motorized wheelchair. You can still walk with the prosthesis when you want to, but you do not have to use up all of your energy just for ambulation. A wheelchair can also be very useful if you are temporarily unable to wear your prosthesis because of poor fit or a skin problem.

Focus on the Positive

Amputees have good days and bad days when living with a prosthesis—whether they are undergoing inpatient rehab or have worn a prosthesis for years. First and foremost, be grateful that you are alive! Focus on how far you have come since you had the amputation. Small steps are most often overlooked, yet they may be the most meaningful. Focus on your achievements: transferring from a bed to a chair, dressing by yourself, bathing yourself, standing for the first time with a prosthesis, walking the length of parallel bars in a rehab gym, driving to get the paper, and playing golf. No matter what you achieve, be proud of the hard work that has gotten you there!

Focus on Small Tasks

Break up complicated tasks into small, easy steps. Instead of worrying about how you are going to walk the length of the parallel bars, worry about taking one step at a time. Focus on shifting your balance from one leg to the other. Concentrate on advancing the prosthetic leg while maintaining your balance on the sound leg. Do not be afraid to ask your therapist for suggestions.

Work toward a Smooth Transition

Going home from the rehab unit may be very stressful for both you and your family, because you are going from a sheltered, attentive environment to one that is more uncertain, and where you will be required to be more independent.

In order to ensure a smooth transition, you may want to ask your rehab therapists to make an advance home visit. They can assess the kitchen, bathrooms, and doorways in your home for any potential risks and make recommendations before you go home.

Confront Your Fears and Find Practical Ways to Overcome Them

There are many fears in living with a prosthesis—fear of falling, fear of being alone, and fear of the loss of independence. Confront your fears head on and try to address them. The fear of falling and not being able to get up is a very common fear for lower limb amputees. Ask your therapist to teach you how to get up off the floor if you fall.

If you are afraid that your spouse or other family members will not be able to take care of you, express this concern honestly. Perhaps your spouse feels that they will not be able to assist in bathing you. Perhaps he/she is worried about leaving you at home by yourself when he/she is at work. Have your spouse visit you during your therapy on the rehab unit. He/she can speak with your therapists in order to relieve any fears he/she may have. It may put your spouse's mind at ease about leaving you alone during the day if he/she sees how well you are doing in your therapy. If bathing is an issue, consider getting a home health attendant to help you.

Another fear might be about returning to work or school. Site visits may be useful in order to see if modifications are needed for you to return to work. If a return to work is not possible, there are various vocational rehab programs that can retrain you to perform your previous job, or retrain you for a new job. Your rehab team can provide you with more information about these options. Again, the key is to be an active, involved participant in your rehabilitation. Try to solve problems as they come up. By being informed, you will expand your options, empower yourself, and become the best advocate for your needs.

Social Etiquette in Difficult Situations

The author has had several patients who experienced the embarrassment of having their prosthetic leg fall off while at a theatre, restaurant, or friend's house. This can be an awkward moment for everyone involved. You should talk to your rehab team and the members of your amputee support group about what to say and do if this happens to you. Some people use humor; others choose to deal with it in a more direct, nonconfrontational way. You have to eventually find a way to be comfortable with your handicap. When you do, others around you will follow your lead. If you are angry, bitter, and resentful about having a prosthesis, the people around you will pick up on it, and everyone will feel awkward.

Find a way to make peace with your loss. When an awkward moment comes, deal with it honestly. Tell your friends and family members that sometimes the leg falls off, and you just have to put it back on. If you deal with it in a comfortable, matter-of-fact, honest way, then everyone concerned will be better off.

Get the Most Out of Your Rehab Team

Remember that your rehab team is there to help you. For the most part, they are practical, open-minded people. Ask them practical, problemfocused questions. You should also be open to their suggestions. An open, honest dialogue is the best way to get your concerns addressed.

Social Support System

One of the most important things that you will need in order to successfully live as an amputee is a good social support system. You will be at a significant disadvantage if you live by yourself, isolated and cut-off from the rest of the world. If you are part of a large, caring family and have many friends, consider yourself lucky, and do not be shy about asking for help. Now is the time to call in those favors and the good will that you have cultivated over the years.

If you have been living alone independently, seek support after discharge from the rehab unit. Join a local amputee support group and go to meetings on a regular basis. Your rehab team can help you find a group in your neighborhood. If one does not exist, then start one yourself. If you do not want to start one, consider volunteering at the rehab unit after discharge to help other amputees cope with their loss. The take-home message is to stay active!

Warning Signs

Difficulty sleeping, poor appetite, weight loss, and feelings that life is not worth living are signs of a potentially more serious underlying depression. Talk to your doctor if you experience any of these symptoms.

Remember the Ultimate Goal—Be Functional, Active, and Enjoy Life!

KEY POINTS

1. There is no right or wrong way to feel after amputation surgery. Your reaction is individual and is shaped by your life experiences.

2. Always ask questions and keep a notebook handy at all times. Remember that rehab is like school, and the rehab professionals are your teachers.

3. Remember that you are lucky to be alive!

4. Develop a good working relationship with at least one of your rehab professionals.

5. Have realistic expectations.

6. Surround yourself with people who care about you. Join or start a support group in your area.

Glossary

AKA: Common term used to describe an above-the-knee amputation. Also referred to as a transfemoral amputation.

Amputee: Term used to describe a person with an amputation.

BKA: Common term used to describe a below-the-knee amputation. Also referred to as a transtibial amputation.

Choke Syndrome: Term given to the appearance of a residual limb in an ill-fitting socket. The top portion of the residual limb is "choked" by the ill-fitting socket, and the lower portion is swollen and red.

Constant Friction Knee: Type of prosthetic knee used in an above-the-knee prosthesis. It is durable, and is indicated for walking primarily on flat surfaces at a single speed.

Contracture: Term used to describe the loss of motion in a joint because of stiffness and tightness of the structures in and around that joint; commonly seen in the hip, knee, and shoulder. A contracture is difficult to reverse once it becomes fixed. It can negatively impact the use of a prosthesis.

Doff: Term used for taking off a prosthesis.

Don: Term used for putting on a prosthesis.

Edema: Swelling caused by retention of fluid in the tissues of the body.

Endoskeletal: Piece of metal that connects the socket of a BKA prosthesis with the foot component. In an AKA prosthesis, this piece connects the knee component with the foot.

Exoskeletal: Type of shank that is made out of a hard shell. It is very durable, but it can be heavy. Once made, it is difficult to adjust.

Energy-Storing Foot: A type of prosthetic foot that is meant to simulate a more normal walking pattern by storing energy when the heel hits the ground, and returning that energy to the foot when the toes push off the ground.

Gait Cycle: Term used to describe the act of walking. It is divided into two phases—stance and swing.

Ischial Containment Socket: Type of socket used in an AKA prosthesis. It is narrower in width than other types of sockets. Its primary advantage is that it provides a good, intimate fit between the thigh muscles and the prosthesis. It also provides good support to the buttocks and pelvic bones.

Neuroma: Nerve trapped inside the scar tissue of the residual limb. It can be a source of pain when wearing a prosthesis.

Phantom Pain: Painful sensation in the region where the amputated limb used to be.

Phantom Sensation: A nonpainful sensation that the amputated limb is still present.

Pistoning: Term used to describe the up and down motion of the residual limb inside a socket that is too big.

Physiatrist: A physician who specializes in rehabilitation medicine and the care of patients with amputated limbs.

Polycentric Knee: Type of prosthetic knee used in the AKA prosthesis, characterized by multiple centers of rotation as it bends. Its main advantage is that it can offer stability during walking.

Prosthesis: Term used to describe artificial limb.

Prosthetist: A rehabilitation professional who designs and fabricates prostheses.

Residual Limb: Term used to describe the remaining part of the amputated limb; commonly known as the *stump.*

SACH Foot (solid ankle cushioned heel): Type of prosthetic foot that has a soft, cushioned heel. It is very durable and is typically prescribed for a sedentary person who does not walk very much.

Shank: The prosthetic component that connects the socket to the foot in the BKA prosthesis, or the knee to the foot in the AKA prosthesis; may be endoskeletal or exoskeletal.

Shrinker: A tight stocking that is worn over the residual limb; helps decrease the swelling that is common after amputation surgery.

Socket: The prosthetic component that surrounds the residual limb and provides an intimate fit.

Stance Phase: The part of walking when the foot is on the ground.

Stump: The term used to describe the part of the limb that is still present after amputation. Also known as the *residual limb.*

Suction Suspension System: A type of suspension used to keep the socket attached to the residual limb. It works on the principle that as the limb is inserted into the prosthesis, air is pushed out through a one-way valve. This creates a negative pressure inside the socket that keeps it suspended from the residual limb. This is a very good type of suspension.

Swing Phase: The part of walking when the foot is not touching the ground.

Syme Amputation: This is an amputation through the ankle region. The advantage of having this type of amputation is that the weight of the body can be directly born on the residual limb. It is not very cosmetic, but it can be very functional.

Vaulting: Term used to describe the raising of the body off the ground by the sound limb. This is done to ensure that the leg with the prosthetic limb does not trip over the floor during the swing phase. Vaulting is usually caused by a prosthesis that is too long, has an ill-fitting socket, or is inadequately suspended from the residual limb.

References

Chapter 1

1. *Footcare: Taking Charge of Your Diabetes.* (Public Service Publication), Roerig, a division of Pfizer Pharmaceuticals.

2. Graham S., Morley M. What "foot care" really means. *Am. J. Nursing* ; 84:889-891; 1984.

3. *The Care and Prevention of Insensitive Feet.* Neville JP, Ed. United States Public Health Services Hospital, Rehabilitation Research Department, Carville, LA.

Chapter 4

4. Smith D. "Notes From the Medical Director: The Knee Disarticulation: It's Better When It's Better and It's Not When It's Not." *inMotion* ; Jan/Feb 2004, pp.56-62.

5. Smith D. "Notes From the Medical Director: The Transformal Amputation Level Part 1: 'Doc, it's 10 times more difficult.'" *inMotion* ; Mar/Apr 2004, pp.54-58.

Chapter 5

6. Rhinestein, J. "The Benefits and Risks of Immediate Post-Operative Prosthesis (IPOP'S)." *inMotion;* Sep/Oct 2003, pp.24-25.

Chapter 7

7. Michael, J.W. "Prosthetic Knee Mechanisms." *Physical Medicine and Rehabilitation. State of the Art Reviews.* Vol.8, No.1, Feb 1994. Philadelphia, PA: Hanley and Belfus Inc.

8. Michael, J.W. "Modern Prosthetic Knee Mechanisms." *Clinical Orthopedics and Related Research.* Number 361. Philadelphia, PA: Lippincott Williams & Wilkins Inc., 1999, pp.39-47.

9. Michael, J.W. "Overview of Prostheses." *Clinical Orthopedics: Orthopedic Rehabilitation.* pp.837-850.

Chapter 8

10. Esquenazi A., Ed. *Prosthetics. State of the Art Reviews.* Vol.8: No.1, Feb.1994. Philadelphia, PA: Hanley and Belfus Inc.

11. Dowell, J. "Don't Forget About the Socket." *inMotion* ; Sep/Oct 2003, pp.10-12.

Chapter 10

12. Alexander A. *Amputee's Guide: Below the Knee.* Issaquah, Washington: Medic Publishing Company, 1975.

Chapter 14

13. Leonard EI, McAnelly RD, Lomba M, et al. "Lower limb prostheses." *Physical Medicine and Rehabilitation, 2nd Ed.* Braddom, RL, Ed. Philadelphia, PA: WB Saunders Co., 2000.

Chapter 16

14. Fordyce D, Trexler LE. "Psychological Perspectives on Rehabilitation: Contemporary Assessment and Intervention Strategies." *Physical Medicine and Rehabilitation, 2nd Ed.* Braddom, RL, Ed. Philadelphia, PA: WB Saunders Co., 2000, pp.75-92.

RESOURCES

Additional Reading

Field Manual for Foot Health. Veterans Health Administration, September 2001.

Muilenberg AC, Wilson AB. *A Manual for Above Knee Amputees.* The American Academy of Orthotists and Prosthetists. Alexandria, Virginia, 1989.

Muilenberg AC, Wilson AB. *A Manual for Below Knee Amputees.* The American Academy of Orthotists and Prosthetists. Alexandria, Virginia, 1991.

Broyles N. *For the New Amputee.* The American Academy of Orthotists and Prosthetists. Alexandria, Virginia, 1991.

Sales C, Goldsmith J, Veith FJ, Eds. *Handbook of Vascular Surgery.* St. Louis, Missouri: Quality Medical Publishing, 1994.

Leonard JA, Meier RH. "Upper and lower extremity prosthetics" in DeLisa J, *Rehabilitation Medicine: Principles and Practice.* Philadelphia, PA: JB Lippincott Company; p.507-525, 1993.

Seymour R. *Prosthetics and Orthotics: Lower Limb and Spinal.* Philadelphia, PA: Lippincott, Williams & Wilkins, 2002.

Organizations

National Center on Physical Activity and Disability (NCPAD), www.ncpad.org.

American Orthotic and Prosthetic Association, www.aopnet.org.

American Academy of Orthotists and Prosthetists, www.oandp.org.

Amputee Coalition of America, www.amputee-coalition.org.

National Family Caregiver Association, www.nf cacares.org.

National Alliance for Caregiving, www.caregivi ng.org.

Back Cover Material

Limb loss can occur due to trauma, infection, diabetes, vascular disease, cancer, and other diseases. Regardless of the cause, it often has a profound impact on a person's life. Many amputees experience feelings of loss and grief, frustration in learning to walk with an artificial limb, and difficulty adjusting to a new and challenging lifestyle. This book provides the practical knowledge needed to cope with the many changes caused by lower limb amputation. In clear, accessible language, it covers the medical, physical, and psychosocial issues and answers crucial questions such as:

- How do I cope emotionally with the loss of a limb?

- What steps can I take to prevent additional amputations?

- How do I treat and care for my post-surgery wound?

- What are the best prostheses for my particular needs?

- Can I play sports and exercise with a prosthesis? And much more!

This unique resource aims to educate those with lower limb amputation so that they can better care for themselves and maximize their independence. The practical advice, tips, and extensive references within its pages will help individuals meet the challenges of leading full and fruitful lives.

About the Author: Dr. Adrian Cristian is Chief of the Department of Rehabilitation Medicine and the Amputee Care Program at the Bronx Veterans Affairs Medical Center, as well as Assistant Professor of Rehabilitation Medicine at the Mount Sinai School of Medicine. He is the author of *Living with Spinal Cord Injury: A Wellness Approach* and the editor of the professional reference, *Aging with a Disability*.

Books For ALL Kinds of Readers

At ReadHowYouWant we understand that one size does not fit all types of readers. Our innovative, patent pending technology allows us to design new formats to make reading easier and more enjoyable for you. This helps improve your speed of reading and your comprehension. Our EasyRead printed books have been optimized to improve word recognition, ease eye tracking by adjusting word and line spacing as well as minimizing hyphenation. Our EasyRead SuperLarge editions have been developed to make reading easier and more accessible for vision-impaired readers. We offer Braille and DAISY formats of our books and all popular E-Book formats.

We are continually introducing new formats based upon research and reader preferences. Visit our web-site to see all of our formats and learn how you can Personalize our books for yourself or as gifts. Sign up to Become A (RHYW) Registered Reader.

www.readhowyouwant.com

LaVergne, TN USA
23 January 2011
213628LV00003B/5/P